"Now with *The I Love Amer*  li-
cally sound method for a l: ht
control and health mainten n-
mend it highly."
> —ALFRED STEINER, M.D., F.A.C.P.
> Emeritus Clinical Professor of Medicine
> College of Physicians and Surgeons
> Columbia University

"Avoiding the bland style of most diet books, Phyllis George and Bill Adler have written a book which is designed for Americans who want to eat properly, look their best, and feel like a million."
> —JAMES A. PETERSON, PH.D.
> Director of Sports Medicine
> Women's Sports Foundation

"*The I Love America Diet* is a sensible and appropriate approach to nutritional change. . . . If the American public adopted this diet, I am convinced that improved health and longevity would result."
> —HAROLD S. SOLOMON, M.D.
> Director, Healthstyle Program
> Harvard Medical School

"The theme of this book departs from the plethora of 'sure-fire' fad diets now available and presents a realistic approach to weight reduction and proper weight maintenance."
> —DR. RUSSELL MOORE
> Assistant Professor of Orthopaedic Surgery
> Johns Hopkins University School of Medicine

The
I ♥
AME
DIET

The I ♥ AMERICA DIET

BY PHYLLIS GEORGE AND BILL ADLER

Based on The Federal Dietary Guidelines for Americans
and official U.S. weight-control recommendations

William Morrow and Company, Inc.
New York   *1983*

Library of Congress Catalog Card Number: 82-51183

ISBN: 0-688-01621-9

Printed in the United States of America

First Edition

1 2 3 4 5 6 7 8 9 10

BOOK DESIGN BY BERNARD SCHLEIFER

THE MOST ACCLAIMED DIET IN AMERICA

What Doctors and Celebrities
Are Saying About

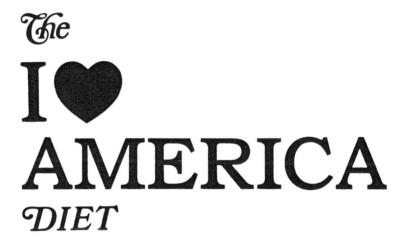

The
I ❤ AMERICA DIET

"Hurrah, a commonsense book based on the recommendations of the nation's best scientific nutritionists and physicians interested in better health through diet.

"A record number of Americans need to change their diet in order to control the diseases of obesity, cancer, diabetes mellitus, and cardiovascular disease. This book provides an excellent diet plan, exercise routine, and new habits required to get started in a safe and effective fashion."
                    —DR. GEORGE L. BLACKBURN
                    Associate Professor of Surgery
                    Chief, Nutrition/Metabolism Laboratory
                    Cancer Research Institute
                    Harvard Medical School

"After all the baloney, we finally have some solid—and nutritious—advice on proper diet. This book is a joy to read and a welcome relief from all the sensational fad diet books that promise so much and deliver so little. Not only is *The I Love America Diet* book factually correct, it is also practical and sensible. It should help millions to reach a weight and physical condition that will add both years and pleasure to their lives."
                    —NORMAN M. KAPLAN, M.D.
                    Professor of Internal Medicine
                    Chief, Hypertension Division
                    University of Texas
                    Health Science Center at Dallas
                    Southwestern Medical School
                    Author of *Prevent Your Heart Attack*

"The authors of this excellent book deserve the highest praise. They have produced the definitive guide to eating sensibly, enjoyably and healthfully.

"*The I Love America Diet* properly advises two of the most important elements of good health—intelligent eating and physical fitness. Its no-nonsense, straightforward, medically sound approach stands in marked contrast to what has been available to the American public until now.

"Not the least of the book's virtues is that it is well organized, a clear presentation, which will contribute greatly to its usefulness."

—DR. JOHN SARNO
Professor Clinical Rehabilitation Medicine
New York University School of Medicine

"At last—a no-nonsense diet tied to exercise in an appropriate manner. Who could tell about it with more enthusiasm than a former Miss America?"

—DR. RALPH E. MINEAR, JR.
Instructor in Pediatrics
Massachusetts General Hospital, Boston

"[*The I Love America Diet*] should serve well as a reference for people at large. Its broadness (diet habits, diet patterns, behavior modification and exercise habits) are those which I personally feel are important in maintaining a healthy body."

—PAUL A. THORNTON, PH.D.
Chairman, Department of Clinical Nutrition
College of Allied Health Professions
University of Kentucky Medical Center

"The content is indeed very applicable to the needs of many Americans today in all walks and stages of life. Your enthusiasm and motivation techniques expressed in the book will

4

convince your reader to make changes in his eating habits and life-style."

—STARR GANTZ, R.D.
Young Parents Program
Department of Obstetrics/Gynecology
University of Kentucky Medical Center

"The theme of this book departs from the plethora of 'sure-fire' fad diets now available and presents a realistic approach to weight reduction and proper weight maintenance."

—DR. RUSSELL MOORE
Assistant Professor of Orthopedic Surgery
Johns Hopkins University
School of Medicine

"For many years I have repeatedly prescribed diets to the same individuals most of which have resulted in a temporary weight loss only to be replaced shortly by a return to the previous overweight status. Now with *The I Love America Diet* an effective, medically sound method for a lifetime program of weight control and health maintenance is available. I recommend it highly."

—ALFRED STEINER, M.D., F.A.C.P.
Emeritus Clinical Professor of Medicine
College of Physicians and Surgeons
Columbia University

"*The I Love America Diet* is a sensible and appropriate approach to nutritional change. The major points of this book are well substantiated and nutritionally and behaviorally correct. If the American public adopted this diet, I am convinced that improved health and longevity would result."

—HAROLD S. SOLOMON, M.D.
Director, Healthstyle Program
Assistant Professor of Medicine
Harvard Medical School

"A sane, sound, reasonable approach to better health at any age. I recommend it without reservations. It represents the best current medical thought without straitjacket rigidity."

—Dr. Leo H. Elstein
Former Borough Chief of Epidemiology
Department of Health
New York City

"*The I Love America Diet* is the prototype of the type of book weight-conscious Americans should be seeking. It explains how proper nutrition can help you lead a more joyful life, why you should be fit, and what steps to follow to achieve nutritionally sound eating habits. Avoiding the bland, boring style of most diet books, Phyllis George and Bill Adler have written a book that is designed for Americans who want to eat properly, look their best, and feel like a million."

—James A. Peterson, Ph.D.
Director of Sports Medicine
Women's Sports Foundation

"A multi-faceted strategy for healthful and sustained weight reduction, which combines sound and achievable dietary practices and an absolutely essential program of enjoyable physical exercise."

—Dr. Ari Kiev
Author of *Strategy
for Daily Living*

"*The I Love America Diet* is easy to read. It should be of considerable assistance to anyone who wants to increase their general health status as well as those who are interested in weight loss through a combination of nutrition and physical activity.

"I especially like your approach whereby the individual is an active participant in organizing his diet patterns. It seems to me that too many of the current diet books require a rote following of iron-clad rules, which must be of diminished usefulness over time."

—FRANCES R. R. DAVIDSON
Assistant Professor
Department of Community and
Family Medicine
School of Medicine,
Georgetown University
Washington, D.C.

"I like the rather breezy style. Dieting should, after all, be an acceptable, challenging part of life—not a grim endurance contest.

"The comparison between scientifically sound and fad diets is well done, and important. Such a comparison is not usually found in diet books.

"There is a good coverage of common dieting problems. I like the 'we are trying to be practical' approach."

—RUTH L. HUENEMANN, D. SC.
Professor Emeritus
Public Health Nutrition Program
University of California,
Berkeley

"*The I Love America Diet* by Phyllis George and Bill Adler is a versatile, sensible, no-nonsense guide to getting slim and staying that way. It shows us not only what foods we should be eating and how much, but also how we should go about eating these foods and when. And it is nutritionally sound.

7

"The comparisons between low-, medium-, and high-calorie versions of specific foods based on their method of preparation are also illuminating. So is the discussion of how our weight is influenced by the way we go about eating—little bites or big bites, slow or fast, with utensils or with fingers, even by how often we brush our teeth and rinse our mouths!

"Dieters will like the formula for estimating how many calories must be taken in to maintain a desirable weight and how many calories must be burned off or subtracted from the diet to lose a given amount of body fat. Such a formula will give dieters a sense of being in charge of their weight destiny.

"And finally, the chapter on exercise, with its focus on how to work out by walking, is a real gem. I have never done warm-up exercises before walking—it never occurred to me to do so. Now I know why my back has so often felt stiff and achy after what I thought was supposed to have been a long 'healthy' walk. No more."

—SALLY WICKLUND, R.N.

"I am a medical innocent and frankly I have been somewhat suspicious of diet books. But also, as a newsman, I know too well how difficult it is to reconcile good eating habits with the demands of a hectic workday. And this book appears to me to provide a practical guide that tackles this very problem."

—WALTER CRONKITE

"Phyllis George and Bill Adler have penned the ultimate diet book. I wholeheartedly endorse this wonderful, sensible and easy-to-follow diet."

—LARRY KING

8

"Ronald Reagan says he is trying to get government 'off our backs.' Phyllis George and Bill Adler, on the other hand, are trying to get Americans off their own lazy backs with the help of such branches of government as the U.S. Department of Agriculture, the U.S. Department of Health and Human Services and the President's Council on Physical Fitness. Their prescription, quite seriously, deserves wide attention.

"Who could possibly argue that most of us eat and exercise properly? The sad fact is, few of us do. This book will help us to shape up, physically and psychologically."

—STEVE ALLEN

"Your measuring cup will become your best friend on this one.

"This diet is definitely not boring. The key is small portions that should satisfy your tummy and your silhouette.

"Try it. You'll be surprised. You'll be satisfied and slim."

—TINA LOUISE

"I have just instructed my lawyer to sue you for thirty million dollars because you have stolen my secret system for remaining slim, energetic, and healthy!

"Seriously, your new *The I Love America Diet* book is filled with just exactly the kind of commonsense advice that I have used to guide me in living the kind of active, on-the-go life that has kept me out of the clutches of doctors and hospitals all my years.

"Every time a new, 'kooky' diet book comes out, I shake my head in despair at the unreasonable hopes of fatties all over the country. I may even start a new television series called 'People Are Funny About Dieting.'

9

"Money, fame, power, and yes, even sex appeal, mean nothing if you don't feel well. I hope that your book will guide millions to a lifetime of feeling their best."

—ART LINKLETTER

"*The I Love America Diet* is so sensible and healthy that it'll blow your fat off."

—SUZY CHAFFEE

"At last a diet that is sensible and sane and works for people of all sizes and shapes."

—WILLARD SCOTT
NBC-TV
Today

"Surprise! Hiding behind a whimsical title, *The I Love America Diet*, and a star-studded cast of authors, George and Adler, is one of the sanest and surest diets ever. As a matter of fact, this book is packed with so much good weight-loss advice that the dieter will want to chain it to the fridge as a lifetime plan."

—JOHN MACK CARTER
Editor-in-Chief
Good Housekeeping

"From cover to cover, *The I Love America Diet* book offers a practical and economical approach to staying healthy. Men and women throughout our great nation should profit from this comprehensive book about diet, exercise and good eating habits. This book not only provides guidelines to follow to maintain physical fitness and well-being, but also it is enjoyable to read and practical to adapt in one's daily routine."

—NANCY THURMOND

"Phyllis George has given us an exercise program that will keep us in shape and a diet program that will help us lose weight."
—GEORGE ALLEN
Chairman of the President's Physical Fitness Council

"Thanks to Phyllis George and Bill Adler, now all Americans can lose weight on *The I Love America Diet*."
—GENE RAYBURN
Television Personality

"As an athlete, I know a good nutritional and exercise program keeps the body finely tuned. As a businessman, I know a good nutritional and exercise program keeps the mind clear and gives one the necessary energy to make it through a hectic day's schedule.

"In this world of new diets, new pills, new exercise programs, it is refreshing to find the plan to help us reach our ideal weight in a healthy and tasty way for a lifetime. *The I Love America Diet* book gets back to the basics and is a 'must' for every home."
—ROGER STAUBACH

"Phyllis George deserves our thanks for a diet that will shape up America."
—FRAN TARKENTON

"For those who can't resist good food but don't want the extra pounds, Phyllis has a hit."
—RUSTY STAUB

"One of the most important factors to a healthy and productive life is a proper diet—and to me that means a well-balanced variety of foods with everything in moderation. With so much attention lately on miracle foods, I'm glad that Phyllis and Bill are getting back to the basics."

—BRUCE JENNER

"The most comprehensive diet I have ever read."

—ED McMAHON

"It will change your life and change your shape—the best diet you could possibly be on. It really works!"

—PAT COLLINS
CBS-TV *Morning News*

"I have known Phyllis George for a long time and I am very impressed but not surprised at the quality of this all-American diet book. As a matter of fact, it was so good I could have eaten it."

—LYNDA CARTER

"To my way of thinking, this is just about the most practical, sensible and enjoyable book on the subject of diet and well-being I have read in a long, long time. I'm going to follow its wise insights for health and energy's sake."

—NORMAN VINCENT PEALE

"When you try this diet
I am sure you'll buy it
all the weigh!"

—SAMMY CAHN
Lyricist

"*The I Love America Diet* gets my vote. It works!"

—ARLENE DAHL

"*The I Love America Diet* will help keep all Americans thin and fit."

—HAL DAVID
Lyricist and President of ASCAP

"This is the most generous of all diets. Imagine—you can eat anything you like, cooked any way you like, and still lose weight healthfully! The best part is, your whole family will love it, too."

—FRANCINE PRINCE
Author of *New Gourmet Recipes for Dieters*

"*The I Love America Diet* will guarantee sensible weight loss, personal well-being, and a more vital and youthful life. As one who has studied nutrition and exercise in detail for over twenty years, I recommend most heartily this common-sense and medically sound approach to weight loss and physical fitness."

—PAT ROBERTSON
President, Christian Broadcasting Network
700 Club Host

"A strong, vital America
depends on
physically fit Americans.
Can we depend on you?"
—*The President's Council
on Physical Fitness and Sports*

SPECIAL THANKS TO:

Dr. Luise Light and Dr. Frances J. Cronin, who are, respectively, Acting Deputy Administrator and Branch Leader, Dietary Guidance Research, Nutrition Guidance and Research Division, Human Nutrition Information, United States Department of Agriculture, for their patience in answering our questions, and supplying us with much of the basic information on which this book is based; and to Paul A. Thornton, Ph.D., and Starr Gantz, R.D., respectively Chairman of the College of Health Professions, Department of Clinical Nutrition, and Director, Young Parents Program, Department of Obstetrics and Gynecology, Albert B. Chandler Medical Center, University of Kentucky, and to Ruth L. Huenemann, D.Sc., Professor Emeritus, Public Health Nutrition Program, University of California, Berkeley, who reviewed the manuscript while it was fresh from the typewriter, and made invaluable contributions.

Our special thanks, too, for their generous assistance goes to Barbara Dennis, M.S., R.D., Nutritionist, Lipid Metabolism-Atherogenesis Branch, Public Health Services, National Institutes of Health, Department of Health and Human Services; Nancy Raper, Home Economist, Consumer Nutrition Center, Human Nutrition Information Service, United States Department of Agriculture; Dr. Ruth N. Klippstein, Extension Faculty Professor, Division of Nutritional Sciences, Cornell University; Dr. Richard O. Keelor, Director of Program Development, The President's Council on Physical Fitness and Sports; Grace L. Ostenso, Science Consultant, Science Research and Technology Subcommittee, Committee on Science and Technology, U.S. House of Representatives; and Norine D. Condon, R.D., Assistant Executive Director, Public Affairs, The American Dietetic Association.

ACKNOWLEDGMENT

*We would like to thank Harold Prince
for his inestimable help
in the preparation of this book.*

Contents

Introduction

HELLO. I'M PHYLLIS GEORGE BROWN. I'm a career woman, a mother, and the wife of Governor John Y. Brown, Jr., of Kentucky.

I created this book with Bill Adler because I wanted to bring you information from United States Government Agencies that could change your life for the better.

It's information about being slim and energetic, about being healthy and fit, about looking wonderful and feeling terrific.

This is not just a diet. It's a complete health program for choosing nutritious foods, adopting new slimming eating habits, and enjoying workouts that shape your body while boosting your stamina and vitality.

This is information that can benefit all of us.

I'm Bill Adler. I'd like to tell you why Phyllis George Brown is the ideal person to bring this good news to you.

As a former Miss America, she *knows* how a complete

29

health program can make you feel your best—and when you feel your best, you look your best.

As network television's first woman sportscaster (Phyllis George is an Emmy Award winner) and a former National Chairperson for Community Affairs for the Special Olympics, she *knows* how a complete health program can stimulate your body to peak performance time after time.

As a recipient of the "Outstanding Mother of the Year Award," she *knows* the importance of a complete health program to keep her family, and herself, in top condition always. She follows the guidelines in this book, and enjoys golf, tennis, horseback riding and going on after-dinner walks with her husband, and especially jumping rope.

And currently, because of her extensive duties as First Lady of Kentucky and chairperson and member of the board of several organizations, she *knows* how a complete health program can keep you going at full speed no matter how hard you have to work. She's doing it.

She *knows*.

Both of us say:

Let's work together to make our country healthier. You owe it to your family and to yourself to give your body the care it deserves. You *can* do it on *The I Love America Diet*. The very best time to start on it is *today*. You'll be giving yourself a gift that could last for the rest of your life.

1

The I Love America Diet: It's Designed for a Lifetime of Slimness and Health

THIS IS A DIET for sensible dieters.

It's a diet for men and women who know that most fad diets *do* work—but only for a short time, never for a lifetime.

It's a diet for people who want to start today to stay slim for the rest of their lives.

It's a diet that becomes a way of life for all your tomorrows—an energetic, healthful way of life.

Because it's not just a diet.

It's a weight/health management plan.

Successful people manage their money, manage their careers, manage their emotions. It's time you began to manage your weight and your health.

On the I Love America Diet, you do it in three ways.

You manage what *you eat.*

You manage how *you eat.*

You manage your physical activity.

We tell you how, based mainly on the recommendations

31

of the U.S. Department of Agriculture, the U.S. Department of Health and Human Services and the President's Council on Physical Fitness and Sports.

HOW YOU CAN BENEFIT FROM THIS DIET

- You can go on a weight-reducing program that, with only slight modifications, becomes a weight-maintenance program. That's the only way most of us can keep it off after we take it off. (On fad diets, about 98 percent of dieters regain their lost weight within a year, because there's no way a fad diet can be transformed satisfactorily into a weight-maintenance program.)

- You can lose up to nine to eleven pounds of *fat*—not water—in one month.* This rate of loss is considered by the medical profession as safe and desirable for most dieters. (On fad diets, the initial weight loss—up to ten pounds a week—is mostly water, which is regained when you return to the kind of food you ordinarily eat.)

- You can choose from a wide variety of supermarket foods that suit your taste and your pocketbook. (Fad diets often demand you eat foods you can't find, can't stomach or can't afford.)

- You can make up your own menus or modify our menus, making it as easy to stay on this diet in most restaurants as it is in your own home. (Eating out consistently on fad diets is virtually impossible.)

*This refers to water not contained in fat tissue, which is about 85 percent water.

- You can avoid counting calories by selecting the right amount of servings from four basic food groups. A *serving* is a specific quantity such as "1 apple," or "½ cup spinach" or "3 ounces of lean beef," and so on. (Some fad diets tell you to avoid counting calories by eating as much as you want of certain foods—a practice that could reinforce your tendency to eat too much of all foods.)

- By selecting the right amount of servings from the four basic food groups, you can also obtain a balanced diet— one that provides virtually all the calories and nutrients, including vitamins and minerals, which you need daily. (Fad diets are often so unbalanced that they produce side effects ranging from the uncomfortable to the dangerous.)

- You can profit from the "new nutrition" that emphasizes less fat, saturated fat, cholesterol, sugar and salt, and more fiber in your diet. The new nutrition is designed to decrease the incidence of obesity, heart disease, diabetes and other nutrition-related diseases; improve general health; and extend our life-spans. (No fad diet is based on the new nutrition.)

- You can learn to modify your recipes to comply with the principles of the new nutrition; or you can follow the simple, delicious recipes based on those principles, prepared for you by U.S. Department of Agriculture nutritionists. (Fad diet recipes do not comply with the principles of the new nutrition, and are notoriously dull.)

- You can learn not only *what* to eat, but *how* to eat—by acquiring new eating habits at the table and *away* from the table that will help you reduce and stay reduced. (Virtually all fad diets ignore this vital aspect of dieting.)

• You can eat more, and still lose weight and keep it off, by taking part regularly in a sport or physical activity that you enjoy and find convenient. (Fad diets simply give lip service to the need for a consistent program of exercise.)

In short, you can benefit at long last from a weight/health management program that rids you of unwanted fat safely and keeps it off surely, while it helps you feel better, more energetic, more alive than ever before.

THE KEYSTONE OF THE I LOVE AMERICA DIET: THE FEDERAL DIETARY GUIDELINES FOR AMERICANS

1. *Maintain ideal weight.*
2. *Eat a variety of foods.*
3. *Avoid too much fat, saturated fat and cholesterol.*
4. *Eat foods with adequate starch and fiber.*
5. *Avoid too much sugar.*
6. *Avoid too much sodium.*
7. *If you drink alcohol, do so in moderation.*

Get acquainted with the following explanation of these guidelines, and you'll understand the "why" of this diet. That will make it easy for you to shape the diet to your own eating preferences and lifestyle.*

1. *Maintain ideal weight.* If you are too fat, your chances of developing some chronic disorders are increased. Obesity is associated with high blood pressure, increased levels of

---

*The material in this section is drawn mainly from *Nutrition and Your Health: Dietary Guidelines for Americans,* published jointly in 1980 by the U.S. Department of Agriculture and the U.S. Department of Health, Education and Welfare (now known as the U.S. Department of Health and Human Services).

blood fats (triglycerides) and cholesterol, and the most common type of diabetes. All of these, in turn, are associated with increased risks of heart attack and strokes. For these compelling reasons, you should try to maintain your ideal weight.

How do you determine what is the ideal weight for you?

There is no absolute answer. The following table shows "acceptable" ranges for most adults. If you have been obese since childhood, you may find it difficult to reach or to maintain your weight within the acceptable range. For most people, their weight should not be more than it was when they were young adults (twenty to twenty-five years old).

SUGGESTED DESIRABLE WEIGHTS[b] AND WEIGHT RANGES

Height[a] in.	MEN lb	WOMEN lb
58	-	102 (92-119)
60	-	102 (96-125)
62	123 (112-141)	113 (102-131)
64	130 (118-148)	113 (102-131)
66	136 (124-156)	128 (114-146)
68	145 (132-166)	136 (122-154)
70	154 (140-174)	144 (130-163)
72	162 (148-184)	152 (138-173)
74	171 (156-194)	-
76	181 (164-204)	-

SOURCE: *Recommended Dietary Allowances*, National Research Council, 1980.
[a] Without shoes.
[b] Without clothes. Average weight ranges in parentheses.

It is not well understood why some people can eat more than others and still maintain normal weight. However, one thing is definite: to lose weight, you must take in fewer calories than you burn. This means you must either select foods containing fewer calories, or increase your physical activity—or both. Good behavioral eating habits will help weight control as well.

To take in fewer calories: Eat less fat, fewer fatty foods, less sugar and fewer sweets, and avoid too much alcohol.

To improve your eating habits: Eat slowly, prepare smaller portions and avoid seconds.

To increase your physical activity: Gradually enter into a regular pattern of exercise that's right for your age and physical condition. Walking, biking and jogging are all good possibilities.

Lose weight gradually. Steady loss of one to two pounds a week—until you reach your goal—is relatively safe and more likely to be maintained. Long-term success depends upon acquiring new and better habits of food selection, eating and exercise.

Do not try to lose weight too rapidly. Avoid crash diets that are severely restricted in the variety of foods they allow. Diets containing fewer than 800 calories may be hazardous. Some people have developed kidney stones, disturbing psychological changes and other complications while following such diets. A few people have died suddenly and without warning.

Do not attempt to reduce your weight below the acceptable range. Severe weight loss may be associated with nutrient deficiencies, menstrual irregularities, infertility, hair loss, skin changes, cold intolerance, severe constipation, psychiatric disturbances and other complications.

2. *Eat a variety of foods.* You need about forty different nutrients to stay healthy. These include vitamins and minerals, as well as amino acids (from proteins), essential fatty acids (from vegetable oils and animal fats*) and sources

---

*Some nutritionists question animal fats as a source of fatty acids in your diet.

of energy (calories from carbohydrates, proteins and fats). These nutrients are in the foods you normally eat.

Most foods contain more than one nutrient. Milk, for example, provides proteins, fats, sugars, riboflavin and other B-vitamins, vitamin A, calcium and phosphorus—among other nutrients.

No single food item supplies all the essential nutrients in the amounts that you need. Milk, for instance, contains very little iron or vitamin C. You should, therefore, eat a variety of foods to assure an adequate diet.

The greater the variety, the less likely you are to develop either a deficiency or an excess of any single nutrient. Variety also reduces your likelihood of being exposed to excessive amounts of contaminants in any single food item.

To assure yourself of an adequate diet: Eat a variety of foods from the following four food groups:

- Fruits and vegetables
- Bread (enriched and whole grain) and cereals. This group includes pasta, grains and other grain products.
- Milk and cheese. This group includes yogurt.
- Meat, fish, poultry and beans. This group includes other legumes and nuts.

There are no known advantages to consuming excess amounts of any nutrient. You will rarely need to take vitamin or mineral supplements if you eat a wide variety of foods.

Exception: Women in their childbearing years may need to take iron supplements to replace the iron they lose with menstrual bleeding. Women who are no longer menstruating should not take iron supplements routinely. Women who are pregnant or who are breast-feeding need more of many nutrients, especially iron, folic acid, vitamin A, calcium and sources of energy (calories from carbohydrates, proteins and fats). And elderly or very inactive people may need dietary supplements. Detailed advice in the use of dietary supplements should come from your physician or from a dietitian.

3. *Avoid too much fat, saturated fat and cholesterol.* If you have a high blood-cholesterol level, you have a greater chance of having a heart attack. Other factors can also increase your risk of heart attack—high blood pressure and cigarette smoking, for example—but high blood cholesterol is clearly a major dietary risk indicator.

Populations like ours with diets high in saturated fats and cholesterol tend to have high blood-cholesterol levels. Individuals within these populations usually have a greater risk of having a heart attack than people eating low-fat, low-cholesterol diets.

Eating extra saturated fat and cholesterol will increase blood-cholesterol levels in most people. However, there are wide variations among people—related to heredity and the way each person's body uses cholesterol.

Some people can consume diets high in saturated fats and cholesterol and still keep normal blood-cholesterol levels. Other people, unfortunately, have high blood-cholesterol levels even if they eat low-fat, low-cholesterol diets.

There is controversy about what recommendations are appropriate for healthy Americans. But for the U.S. population *as a whole,* reduction in our current intake of total fat, saturated fat and cholesterol is sensible. This suggestion is especially appropriate for people who have high blood pressure or who smoke.

The recommendations are not meant to prohibit the use of any specific food item or to prevent you from eating a variety of foods. For example, eggs and organ meats (such as liver) contain cholesterol, but they also contain many essential vitamins and minerals, as well as protein. Such items can be eaten in moderation, as long as your overall cholesterol intake is not excessive. If you prefer whole milk to skim milk, you can reduce your intake of fats from foods other than milk.

To avoid too much fat, saturated fat and cholesterol:

- Choose lean meat, fish, poultry, dry beans and peas as your protein sources.

- Moderate your use of eggs and organ meats (such as liver).

- Limit your intake of butter, cream, hydrogenated margarines, shortenings and coconut oil, and foods made from such products.

- Trim excess fat off meats.

- Broil, bake or boil rather than fry.

- Read labels carefully to determine both the amount and types of fat contained in foods.

4. *Eat foods with adequate starch and fiber.* The major sources of energy in the average U.S. diet are carbohydrates and fats. (Proteins and alcohol also supply energy, but to a lesser extent.) If you limit your fat intake, you should increase your calories from carbohydrates to supply your body's energy needs.

In trying to reduce your weight to "ideal" levels, carbohydrates have an advantage over fats: Carbohydrates contain less than half the number of calories per ounce than fats, so you can replace fatty foods with a greater quantity of carbohydrate foods and still lose weight.

Complex-carbohydrate foods—starchy foods—are better than *simple* carbohydrates in this regard. Simple carbohydrates—such as sugars—provide calories but little else in the way of nutrients. Complex-carbohydrate foods—such as beans, peas, nuts, seeds, fruits* and vegetables, and whole-grain breads, cereals and products—contain many essential nutrients in addition to calories.

Increasing your consumption of certain complex carbohydrates can also help increase dietary fiber. The average American diet is relatively low in fiber. Eating more foods high in fiber tends to reduce the symptoms of chronic constipation, diverticulosis and some types of "irritable bowel." There is also concern that low-fiber diets might increase the risk of developing cancer of the colon, but whether this is true is not yet known.

To make sure you get enough fiber in your diet, you should eat fruits and vegetables, whole-grain breads and cereals. There is no reason to add fiber to foods that do not already contain it.

To eat more complex carbohydrate foods:

• Substitute starches for fats and sugars.

• Select foods that are good sources of fiber and starch, such as whole-grain breads and cereals, fruits and vegetables, beans, peas and nuts.

5. *Avoid too much sugar.* The major health hazard from eating too much sugar is tooth decay (dental caries).† The risk of caries is not simply a matter of how much sugar you eat. The risk increases the more frequently you eat sugar and sweets, especially if you eat between meals, and if you eat foods that stick to the teeth. For example, frequent snacks of sticky candy, or dates, or daylong use of soft drinks may be more harmful than adding sugar to your morning cup of coffee—at least as far as your teeth are concerned.

---

*Fruits may also be regarded as a rich source of simple carbohydrates. (Source: *Nutrition and Diet Therapy*, Sue Rodwell Williams, 4th Edition, The C.V. Mosby Co., St. Louis.)

†For other objections to sugar see page 70.

Obviously, there is more to healthy teeth than avoiding sugars. Careful dental hygiene and exposure to adequate amounts of fluoride in the water are especially important.

Contrary to widespread opinion, too much sugar in your diet does not seem to cause diabetes. The most common type of diabetes is seen in obese adults; and avoiding sugar, without correcting the overweight, will not solve the problem. There is also no convincing evidence that sugar causes heart attacks or blood-vessel diseases.

Estimates indicate that Americans use on the average more than 130 pounds of sugars and sweeteners a year. This means the risk of tooth decay is increased not only by the sugar in the bowl, but also by the sugars and syrups in jams, jellies, candies, cookies, soft drinks, cakes and pies, as well as sugars found in products such as breakfast cereals, catsup, flavored milks and ice cream. Frequently, the ingredient label will provide a clue to the amount of sugars in a product.

To avoid excessive sugar:

- Use less of all sugars, including white sugar, brown sugar, raw sugar, honey and syrups.

- Eat less of foods containing these sugars, such as candy, soft drinks, ice cream, cakes, cookies.

- Select fresh fruits or fruits canned without sugar, or with light syrup rather than heavy syrup.

- Read food labels for clues on sugar content—if the names sucrose, glucose, maltose, dextrose, lactose, fructose or syrups appear first, then there is a large amount of sugar.

- Remember, how often you eat sugar is as important as how much sugar you eat.

6. *Avoid too much sodium.* Table salt contains sodium and chloride—both are essential elements.

Sodium is also present in many beverages and foods that we eat, especially in certain processed foods, condiments, sauces, pickled foods, salty snacks and sandwich meats. Baking soda, baking powder, monosodium glutamate (MSG), soft drinks and even many medications (many antacids, for instance) contain sodium.

It is not surprising that adults in the United States take in much more sodium than they need.

The major hazard of excessive sodium is for persons who have high blood pressure. Not everyone is equally susceptible. In the United States, approximately 17 percent of adults have high blood pressure. Sodium intake is but one of the factors known to affect blood pressure. Obesity, in particular, seems to play a major role.

In populations with a low-sodium intake, high blood pressure is rare. In contrast, in populations with a high-sodium intake, high blood pressure is common. If people with high blood pressure severely restrict their sodium intake, their blood pressure will *usually* fall—although not always to normal levels.

At present, there is no good way to predict who will develop high blood pressure, though certain groups, such as blacks, have a higher incidence. Low-sodium diets might help some of these people avoid high blood pressure if they could be identified before they develop the condition.

Since most Americans eat more sodium than is needed, consider reducing your sodium intake. Use less table salt. Eat sparingly those foods to which large amounts of sodium have been added. Remember that up to half of sodium intake may be "hidden," either as part of the naturally occurring food or, more often, as part of a preservative or flavoring agent that has been added.

To avoid too much sodium:

• Learn to enjoy the unsalted flavors of foods.

• Cook with only small amounts of added salt.

- Add little or no salt to food at the table.

- Limit your intake of salty foods, such as potato chips, pretzels, salted nuts and popcorn, condiments (soy sauce, steak sauce, garlic salt), cheese, pickled foods, cured meats.

- Read food labels carefully to determine the amounts of sodium in processed foods and snack items.

7. *If you drink alcohol, do so in moderation.* Alcoholic beverages tend to be high in calories and low in other nutrients. Even moderate drinkers may need to drink less if they wish to achieve ideal weight.

On the other hand, heavy drinkers may lose their appetite for foods containing essential nutrients. Vitamin and mineral deficiencies occur commonly in heavy drinkers—in part, because of poor intake, but also because alcohol alters the absorption and use of some essential nutrients.

Heavy drinking may also cause a variety of serious conditions, such as cirrhosis of the liver and some neurological disorders. Cancer of the throat and neck is much more common in people who drink and smoke than in people who don't.

One or two drinks daily appear to cause no harm in adults. Selections from a fifth food group—fats, sweets and alcohol—may be made cautiously. Remember, these foods provide calories but few nutrients. If you drink, you should do so in moderation.

HOW TO USE THIS BOOK

The wisest way is to read it through once carefully. That will answer virtually all of your questions, and firm down in your mind the "whys" and the "hows" of the diet. You're then ready to begin to shed pounds.

But before you do, consult with your physician. That's mandatory whenever you change your diet or the degree and/or type of your physical activity. While you're making these changes, do visit your doctor periodically. Everybody is different, and no one can predict how even the safest of diet/exercise plans will affect an individual. Medical surveillance is a prudent precautionary measure for dieters.

If you're ailing, don't look to this diet as a cure-all. It's meant for healthy adults only. No diet can *guarantee* health or well-being. Health depends on many things in addition to diet, including heredity, lifestyle, personality traits, mental health and attitude, and environment. Food *alone*, no matter how good it is for you, cannot make you healthy.

But a combination of a variety of the right foods eaten in moderation, good eating habits and a suitable level of physical activity can help keep you healthy and even improve your health.

That's the message of the Federal Dietary Guidelines for Americans. It's a message from the devoted men and women—legislators and scientists—who conceived the Guidelines and made them available to all of us. It's a message from people who love America, who possess a fervent desire to help most Americans manage their weight and health, so they can live more vigorously and longer, and contribute more to the strength and growth of our magnificent nation. That's why we call our diet, based on the Guidelines and related works, The I Love America Diet. It's a diet for most adult Americans who are concerned about their own well-being and the well-being of the nation—and want to do something about it. After all, it's patriotic to be healthy.

2

The Reducing Diet Menus for Most Women (and Small-Frame Men)

THESE MENUS ARE based on the 1,200-calorie-a-day menu suggested by the Consumer and Food Economics Institute of the U.S. Department of Agriculture.* Jane E. Brody, the Personal Health columnist of *The New York Times*, points out that on the Institute's 1,200-calorie diet, "many people would lose a fair bit of weight." As a matter of fact, since 1958 the Bureau of Nutrition, New York City Department of Health, has been offering a 1,200-calorie *reducing* diet for "most women and small-frame men" that is nutritionally similar to the Institute's diet. This 1,200-calorie reducing diet is designed to produce a fat loss—not water loss—of about 9 to 11 pounds a month (about 2 to 2½ pounds a week).†

---

*It is not regarded by the Institute as a reducing diet, but rather as a basic maintenance diet that can "provide adequate protein, and supply most of the vitamins and minerals you need daily." The Institute advises you to "plan your day's food around this foundation to keep . . . on the right track to a better diet."

†At this rate of fat lost, you consume 1,000 to 1,250 calories a day less than your stay-fat intake. The heavier you are, the more weight you'll lose, and vice versa.

45

The basic 1,200-calorie-a-day menu published by the Institute appears on Day 1 of the I Love America Diet. The menus on Days 2 through 7 were created by us following the Institute's Guidelines.*

However, you are not locked in to any of these menus. By following government guidelines, you can plan your own menus (Chapter 6, page 93). And, on the basis of taste, convenience or cost, you can draw on a great variety of foods to make substitutions (pages 94–107).

You'll find these fat-shedding menus of familiar foods as nutritious as they are appealing to the palate and the eye.

*These Guidelines appear in *Food*, published by the U.S. Department of Agriculture, Science and Education Administration, Human Nutrition Center, Consumer and Food Economics Institute.

THE REDUCING DIET MENUS FOR MOST WOMEN (AND SMALL-FRAME MEN)

Day 1

BREAKFAST
- ½ cup orange juice
- ½ cup bran flakes with raisins
- ½ cup whole milk (we prefer skim, fortified)
- 1 slice whole-wheat toast
  coffee, tea or water

LUNCH
(You can brown-paper-bag this one)
- 1 ham sandwich,* consisting of:
  - 2 ounces ham
  - 1 slice (1 ounce) cheese
  - lettuce
  - ½ medium tomato
  - 2 slices enriched bread
- 1 medium apple
  coffee, tea or water

DINNER
- 3 ounces roast beef
- 1 medium baked potato
- ½ cup broccoli
- 1 cup skim milk, fortified

SNACKS
- 1 small cucumber, sliced
- 3–4 strips carrot (strips are about 2½ to 3 inches long)

*If you're watching your salt intake carefully, you can switch to any unsalted meat (turkey or roast beef, for example).

Day 2

BREAKFAST

- ½   grapefruit
- 1   medium egg, soft cooked
- ½   English muffin
- 1   cup skim milk, fortified
       coffee, tea or water

LUNCH

(You can brown-paper-bag this one)

- 1   tuna fish sandwich, consisting of:
  - 2 ounces canned tuna, packed in water, sprinkled with
  - lemon juice and 1 tablespoon chopped onion
  - 2 slices whole-wheat bread
- 1½ cups tossed salad (suggested ingredients: lettuce, tomato, carrots, green onions)
- 1   medium pear
- 1   1-inch cube natural Cheddar cheese

DINNER

- 2½ ounces broiled lamb chop, lean
- 8   medium asparagus stalks, fresh
- ½   cup green peas
- ½   cup white rice, enriched, steamed or boiled
- ½   cup pineapple, packed in own juice
       coffee, tea or water

SNACK

- ½   cup bean sprouts, or
- ½   cup radishes

Day 3

BREAKFAST
- ½ cup strawberries, fresh or frozen, unsweetened, with
- ½ cup cottage cheese, dry-curd, skim milk, less than .5 percent milk fat, no salt added
- ½ cup cooked cereal of your choice
- 1 cup skim milk, fortified

  coffee, tea or water

LUNCH

(You can brown-paper-bag this one)
- 1 chicken sandwich, consisting of:
  - 2 ounces chicken, preferably white meat
  - 2 slices whole-wheat bread
- 1½ cups mixed green salad (suggested ingredients: spinach, iceberg lettuce, green onions and cucumber) with
- 2 teaspoons Italian dressing
- 1 medium banana

  coffee, tea or water

DINNER
- 2½ ounces broiled cod cooked with margarine, soft
- 1 cup cauliflower, fresh or frozen
- 1 cup green beans, fresh or frozen
- ½ cup noodles
- 1 raisin-walnut delight, consisting of:
  - 1 tablespoon raisins
  - 5 halves shelled walnuts
  - 1 ounce natural Swiss cheese

  coffee, tea or water

SNACK
- ½ tangerine, or
- ½ cup mushrooms, chopped

Day 4

BREAKFAST
- 1   medium orange
- 1   medium egg, scrambled
- 1   small bagel, with
- 1   teaspoon margarine, soft
- 1   cup skim milk, fortified
  coffee, tea or water

LUNCH
(You can brown-paper-bag this one)
- 1   cup tomato juice, preferably with no salt added
- 1   salmon salad, consisting of:
  - 2 ounces canned salmon, packed in water, served on a platter, with
  - 1½ cups combined Romaine lettuce, watercress and sliced radishes, and
  - 2 teaspoons Italian dressing
- 2   slices whole-wheat bread
- ¼   medium cantaloupe
  coffee, tea or water

DINNER
- 1   cup fresh fruit cup (suggested ingredients: slices of banana and apple, grapes and orange sections)
- 3   ounces roast chicken, preferably white meat
- ½   cup lima beans, fresh
- ½   cup spaghetti, enriched, with tomato sauce
- 1   1-inch cube natural Swiss cheese
  coffee, tea or water

SNACKS
- ½   cup broccoli, cooked or raw
- ½   cup cauliflower, cooked or raw

Day 5

BREAKFAST
- ½ cup mixed orange and grapefruit sections
- 2 ounces American cheese
- 1 slice whole-wheat toast
  coffee, tea or water

LUNCH
- 6 medium shrimps, broiled
- 1 pita bread, or 2 slices whole-wheat bread
- 1½ cups mixed green salad (suggested ingredients: spinach, iceberg lettuce, green onions and cucumbers)
- ½ cup vanilla yogurt, with
- ½ cup pineapple chunks, canned, in own juice
  coffee, tea or water

DINNER
- 3 ounces meat loaf
- 1 cup cooked cabbage
- ½ cup beans or peas of your choice
- ½ cup macaroni, without sauce
- 1 cup ice milk, any flavor, with
- ½ cup berries of your choice
  coffee, tea or water

SNACK
- ½ orange, or
- ½ apple

Day 6

BREAKFAST
- ½ cup tomato juice, canned, preferably with no salt added
- ¾ cup ready-to-eat cereal, not presweetened, with
- 1 cup skim milk, fortified
- 1½ teaspoons peanut butter on
- 2 squares graham crackers
  coffee, tea or water

LUNCH
- 1 cheeseburger, consisting of:
  - 2 ounces ground beef, lean
  - 1 ounce American cheese
  - 1 hamburger bun, enriched
- ½ cup coleslaw, preferably made with mayonnaise-type dressing
- 1 small peach
  coffee, tea or water

DINNER
- 1½ cups tossed salad (suggested ingredients: lettuce, tomato, carrots, green onions), with
- 1 tablespoon Italian dressing
- 3 ounces broiled flounder or scrod fillet cooked with margarine, soft
- ½ cup corn
- ½ cup spinach
- ½ cup grapes, with
- 1 1-inch cube natural Cheddar cheese
  coffee, tea or water

SNACKS
- ½ medium cantaloupe
- ½ cup strawberries, unsweetened

Day 7

BREAKFAST
- ½ medium cantaloupe
- 1 average corn muffin, with
- 1 teaspoon jam
- 1 cup skim milk, fortified
  coffee, tea or water

LUNCH
- 1 sardine sandwich, consisting of:
  - 2 ounces sardines
  - lemon juice
  - 2 slices whole-wheat bread
- 1½ cups mixed green salad (suggested ingredients: spinach, iceberg lettuce, green onions and cucumber), with
- 2 teaspoons Italian dressing
- ½ cup berries of your choice, over
- 1 cup cottage cheese, dry-curd, skim milk, less than .5 percent milk fat, no salt added
  coffee, tea or water

DINNER
- ½ cup split-pea soup, canned or homemade
- 2 ounces broiled sirloin steak
  small onion, raw, sliced
- ½ cup broccoli
- ½ cup spinach
- ¾ cup ice milk, any flavor, with
- ½ cup strawberries, fresh or frozen, unsweetened)

SNACKS
- 4 ounces grapefruit or orange juice, fresh or frozen, or
- ½ cup celery, chopped, and
- ½ cup green pepper, chopped

3

The Reducing Diet Menus for Most Men (and Large-Frame Women)

THIS 1,600-CALORIE-A-DAY diet was developed by the Science and Education Administration/Human Nutrition of the U.S. Department of Agriculture.* Jane E. Brody, the Personal Health columnist of *The New York Times*, points out that on this 1,600-calorie diet "many people would lose a fair bit of weight." As a matter of fact, since 1968 the Bureau of Nutrition, New York City Department of Health, has been offering a 1,600-calorie reducing diet for "most men and large-frame women" that is nutritionally similar to the Science and Education Administration/Human Nutrition's diet. This 1,600-calorie reducing diet is designed to produce a fat loss—not a water loss—of almost 9 to 11 pounds a month (about 2 to 2½ pounds a week).†

The menus in this chapter are those created by the nutritionists of the Science and Education Administration.‡ We

---

*It is not intended by that Administration as a reducing diet. Rather, it reflects the amount of food non-dieting women say they eat, on the average, as reported in surveys.

†See footnote page 45.

‡These menus appear in *Ideas for Better Eating: Menus and Recipes to Make Use of the Dietary Guidelines*, published by Science and Education Administration/ Human Nutrition, U.S. Department of Agriculture.

54

have made a few minor changes, mainly to eliminate the need to follow any recipes but your own; but if you would like to try the tested recipes suggested by the nutritionists who created the menus, by all means do so. (Where we've made changes, we've indicated page references to the recipes we've replaced.)

However, you are not locked in to any of these menus. By following government guidelines, you can plan your own menus (Chapter 6, page 93) and, on the basis of taste, convenience or cost, you can draw on a great variety of foods to make substitutions (pages 94–107).

These menus were developed not only with nutritional values in mind, but to keep your dieting appealing and enjoyable as well as healthful.

THE REDUCING DIET MENUS FOR MOST MEN (AND LARGE-FRAME WOMEN)

Day 1

BREAKFAST
- ¾ cup orange juice, fresh or frozen
- 2 slices whole-wheat toast (1)
- ½ cup skim milk, fortified
  coffee, tea or water

LUNCH

(You can brown-paper-bag this one)
- 1 tuna salad sandwich, consisting of:
  - 2 ounces canned tuna, packed in water
  - 1 tablespoon chopped celery
  - 1 teaspoon chopped onion
  - 2 teaspoons mayonnaise
  - 2 slices whole-wheat bread
- 1 medium pear, fresh
- 1 cup skim milk, fortified
  coffee, tea or water

DINNER
- 4 ounces pot roast, chuck, lean only
- ¾ cup mashed potatoes
- ½ cup green beans, fresh or frozen
- 1 cup spinach salad, with
- 1 tablespoon Italian dressing
- 1 slice Italian bread, enriched, with
- 1 teaspoon margarine, soft
- 1 cup mixed orange sections, fresh, and canned pineapples in own juice (2)
  coffee, tea or water

SNACK
1   cup raw sticks of carrot, celery and green pepper, with
¼   cup bean dip, consisting of:
- ¼ can kidney beans, drained, with
- spices to taste, mixed in blender (3)

coffee, tea or water

Alternates:
(1) See recipe for Banana-Nut Bread, page 180.
(2) See recipe for Orange-Pineapple Cup, page 169.
(3) See recipe for Chili Bean Dip, page 222.

Day 2

BREAKFAST
½   cup strawberries, fresh or frozen, unsweetened
2   shredded wheat biscuits, with
1   sliced banana, and
1   cup low-fat milk (2 percent), fortified
coffee, tea or water

LUNCH
1   small hamburger, consisting of:
- 2 ounces ground beef
- hamburger bun, enriched

½   cup coleslaw, with mayonnaise-type dressing
1   small serving french fries
8   ounces fruit or vegetable juice (1)
coffee, tea or water

DINNER
½   cup chicken breast, any style (2)
½   cup spaghetti, enriched
½   cup cooked fresh zucchini

1½ cups mixed green salad (suggested ingredients:
      spinach, iceberg lettuce, green onions and
      cucumbers), with
1   tablespoon Italian dressing
1   slice Italian bread, enriched, with
1   teaspoon margarine, soft
      coffee, tea or water

SNACKS
½   cup low-fat milk (2 percent), fortified
1   medium tangerine

Alternates:
(1) For list of alternates, see page 106.
(2) See recipe for Chicken Cacciatore, page 221.

Day 3

BREAKFAST
¾   cup orange juice, fresh or frozen
1   bagel, with
1   tablespoon cream cheese
1   cup skim milk, fortified
      coffee, tea or water

LUNCH
(You can brown-paper-bag this one)
1   sliced chicken sandwich, consisting of:
      • 2 ounces sliced chicken
      • 1 leaf lettuce
      • 2 teaspoons mayonnaise-type salad dressing
      • 2 slices whole-wheat bread
½   cup bean salad, consisting of:
      • ¼ cup each canned kidney and garbanzo beans,
        drained, mixed together, and garnished with

   • chopped onion and very thinly sliced carrot strips
     to taste
coffee, tea or water

DINNER
1 cup vegetable soup, canned, made with added skim
   milk instead of water (1)
2½ ounces baked cod, sprinkled with 1 tablespoon each
   chopped onion and green pepper (2)
½ cup broccoli spears, fresh or frozen
½ cup brown rice
1½ cups mixed green salad (suggested ingredients:
   spinach, iceberg lettuce, green onion and
   cucumbers), with
1 tablespoon French dressing
½ cup grapes, seedless
   coffee, tea or water

SNACK
1 slice gingerbread (3)

Alternates:
(1) See recipe for Vegetable Chowder, page 175.
(2) See recipe for Spicy Baked Fish, page 222.
(3) See recipe for Gingerbread, page 191.

Day 4

BREAKFAST
¼ medium cantaloupe
1 large egg, soft cooked
1 average corn muffin
½ cup low-fat milk (1 percent), fortified
   coffee, tea or water

LUNCH

(You can brown-paper-bag this one)

1   ham and cheese sandwich, consisting of:
- 1 ounce lean ham
- 1 ounce natural Swiss cheese
- 2 teaspoons mayonnaise-type salad dressing
- 1 leaf lettuce
- 2 slices rye bread

1¼ cups tossed salad (suggested ingredients: lettuce, tomato, carrots, green onions), with
1   tablespoon Italian dressing
1   medium orange
    coffee, tea or water

DINNER

3   ounces broiled flounder fillet sprinkled with 1 tablespoon each chopped onions and Parmesan cheese, served over } (1)
1   cup cooked spinach, fresh or frozen
1   medium baked potato, with
2   tablespoons sour cream
½   cup green peas, frozen
1   small whole-wheat roll, with
1   teaspoon margarine, soft
4   ounces low-fat vanilla yogurt, mixed with
½   cup strawberries, fresh or frozen, unsweetened
    coffee, tea or water

SNACK

1   English muffin, enriched, with
1   tablespoon marmalade

Alternate:

(1) See recipe for Flounder Florentine, page 219.

Day 5

BREAKFAST
- ½   medium grapefruit, fresh
- 2   slices whole-wheat toast, with
- 1   teaspoon margarine, soft
- 1   cup skim milk, fortified
      coffee, tea or water

LUNCH
(You can brown-paper-bag this one)
- ¾   cup tomato juice, canned, preferably with no salt
      added
- 1   luncheon salad, consisting of:
  - 1½ cups mixed greens
  - 1½ ounces natural Swiss cheese
  - 1 tablespoon French dressing
- 1   slice corn bread (1)
- 1   small peach, fresh
      coffee, tea or water

DINNER
- 4   ounces broiled ground beef, lean
- ½   cup corn, fresh or frozen
- ½   cup green beans, fresh or frozen
- 1   baked apple, with
- 2   teaspoons brown sugar
      coffee, tea or water

SNACKS
- 3   squares graham crackers
- 1   cup fruit or vegetable juice (2)

Alternates:
(1) See recipe for Corn Bread, page 189.
(2) For list of alternates, see page 106.

Day 6

BREAKFAST

¾ cup orange juice, fresh or frozen

2 pancakes, prepared mix or homemade, whole-wheat preferred (1), topped with

2 teaspoons blueberry preserve, made with sugar or honey (2)

1 cup low-fat milk (1 percent), fortified

LUNCH

1 supercheeseburger (3), consisting of:
   - 2 ounces ground beef, lean
   - ½ ounce natural sharp Cheddar cheese
   - 1 tablespoon chopped onion
   - 2 tomato slices
   - 2 leaves lettuce
   - 1 hamburger bun

¾ cup fresh fruit cup, consisting of: orange sections, and apple and banana slices

½ cup low-fat milk (1 percent), fortified

DINNER

4 ounces roast loin of pork, lean only

1 small sweet potato, baked

½ cup cooked collard greens, fresh or frozen

1¼ cups tossed salad (suggested ingredients: lettuce, tomato, carrots, green onions), with

1 tablespoon Italian dressing

1 biscuit, enriched, with

1 teaspoon margarine, soft
   coffee, tea or water

SNACKS

4 squares graham crackers

8 ounces fruit or vegetable juice (4)

Alternates:
(1) See recipe for Whole-Wheat Pancakes, page 182.
(2) See recipe for Blueberry Sauce, page 172.
(3) See recipe for Beef Tacos, page 208.
(4) For list of alternates, see page 106.

Day 7

BREAKFAST
- ½   cup pineapple chunks, packed in own juice
- ½   cup oatmeal with cinnamon
- 1   teaspoon brown sugar
- ½   cup low-fat milk (1 percent), fortified
     coffee, tea or water

LUNCH
- 1   cup split-pea soup, canned (1)
- 1   chicken salad stuffed tomato, consisting of:
  - 2 ounces cooked chopped chicken
  - 1 tablespoon chopped celery
  - 1 teaspoon chopped onion
  - 2 teaspoons mayonnaise
  - 1 medium tomato
- 3   rye crackers
     coffee, tea or water

DINNER
- 3   ounces beef, round steak, lean, sautéed
- ½   cup Chinese-style vegetables, canned or frozen } (2)
- ½   cup white rice, enriched
- ¾   cup apple brown betty, preferably made with
     enriched bread; or small slice apple pie (3)
     coffee, tea or water

SNACKS

2   small bananas
2   tablespoons chopped walnuts ⎫
4   squares graham crackers   ⎬ (4)
                                  ⎭
1   medium orange
1   cup low-fat milk (1 percent), fortified

Alternates:

(1) See recipe for Split-Pea Soup, page 202.

(2) See recipe for Beef with Chinese-Style Vegetables, page 220.

(3) See recipe for Apple Crisp, page 173.

(4) See recipe for Banana-Nut Bread, page 180. Two slices are recommended.

4

Answers to Your Questions About The I Love America Reducing Diets

Must I follow the menus exactly as written?

Of course not. The menus guide you to the kinds and amounts of foods that make up a nutritive diet, but you can make choices to fit your eating styles and needs. In Chapter 6, you'll learn how to make up your own menus, and on pages 94–107 you'll discover how to make substitutions in the suggested menus. But if you find it more convenient to follow the menus as they appear, by all means do so.

I've been told to stay away from most canned products because they're high in salt. Why are they on your menus?

Because we're realistic. Most of us like to cut down on our cooking chores, and canned goods are fast and easy. Besides, it's not the amount of salt in one dish that counts, it's the amount you consume in a day. On our daily menus, there's never more salt than the amount recommended by the National Research Council (1,100 to 3,300 milligrams of sodium a day, equivalent to about 2,750 to 8,250 milligrams of salt).

When am I permitted to snack?

It's not a question of "permission." This is your life, and you can live it the way that suits you. When do *you* like to snack? In midmorning? In midafternoon? At TV-time? At bedtime? At other times? *You* decide when to snack, and enjoy it.

Must I eat all my snack food at one time?

If you can stretch out the amount allotted for more than one snack time, great. But, realistically, there isn't that much food to snack on, so your snacks are mostly the one-a-day kind. If you like more than one snack a day, cut down on the calories you consume at one or more of your major meals. On the Man's Diet, Day 7, we've done just that (dinner is light), offering you several snacks you can consume at different times.

Some menus include skim milk, others low-fat (1 percent fat) milk, and still others low-fat (2 percent fat) milk. Why aren't you consistent?

When skim milk is fortified (with vitamins A and D), it has essentially the same nutrients as whole milk (3.5 percent fat), but far less fat (under 1 percent) and far fewer calories. Skim milk makes good sense to a dieter. But if you're accustomed to whole milk, skim milk can be a disappointment. It lacks creaminess. So, to satisfy your taste buds, we suggest you cut down on milk fats and calories by buying low-fat milk, either the 2-percent or the 1-percent fat varieties.

I don't care much for skim milk. May I substitute low-fat milk?

Yes, if you just cut down a bit on the portion sizes of the rest of the meal. But once you get accustomed to skim milk, you'll find it a pleasant, refreshing, thirst-quenching drink with a "clean" taste. Skim-milk fans find even 1 percent low-fat milk sufficiently creamy.

May I use no-fat milk?

If you like it, and it's fortified, of course. The calorie difference between skim and no-fat milk is minor, but there is a taste difference. We find nonfat milk made from "non-instant" dry solids the most pleasing to the palate.

You call for American, Swiss, cottage and Cheddar cheese. That's all?

Of course not. One of the outstanding advantages of the I Love America Diet is that you can enjoy a great variety of foods. Here are some interesting statistics on cheese that could help you make your choice:

COMPOSITION OF SELECTED CHEESES[1]

Cheese	IN ONE OUNCE		
	Calories	Fat[2]	Sodium[3]
American, Cheese Food, Cold Pack	94	6.93	274
Blue	100	8.15	396
Brick	64	5.10	159
Brie	95	7.85	176
Camembert	85	6.88	239
Caraway	107	8.28	196
Cheddar	114	9.40	176
Cheshire	110	8.68	198
Colby	68	5.52	104
Cottage			
Creamed	117	5.10	457

[1] Information derived, except where noted, from *Agriculture Handbook No. 8–1,* published by United States Department of Agriculture, Agriculture Research Service.

[2] In grams.

[3] In milligrams.

IN ONE OUNCE

Cheese	Calories	Fat	Sodium
Dry-curd	96	.48	14
Low-fat (2 percent)	101	2.18	459
Low-fat (1 percent)	82	1.15	459
Dry-curd, skim-milk, less than .5 percent milk fat, no salt added[4]	23	.26	84
Cream	99	9.89	84
Edam	101	7.88	274
Feta	75	6.03	316
Fontina	110	8.83	UK
Gjetost	132	8.37	170
Gouda	101	7.78	232
Gruyère	117	9.17	95
Limburger	93	7.72	227
Monterey	106	8.58	152
Mozzarella	80	6.12	106
Low-moisture	56	4.31	73
Part-skim	72	4.51	132
Low-moisture, part-skim	49	3.01	93
Muenster	104	8.52	178
Neufchâtel	74	6.64	113
Parmesan			
Grated	129	8.51	528
Hard	111	7.32	454
Port du Salut	100	8.00	151
Processed cheese, pasteurized			
American	106	8.75	400
American, cheese spread	82	6.02	381
Pimento	106	8.74	400
Swiss	94	7.01	383
Provolone	100	7.55	248
Ricotta			
Whole-milk	49	3.64	29
Part-skim-milk	39	2.22	35
Romano	110	7.64	340
Roquefort	105	8.69	513
Swiss	105	7.69	73
Tilsit	96	7.36	213

[4] Manufacturer's statistics.

Sometimes you specify "toast" and sometimes just "bread." Why?

Let's make one thing clear: We don't "specify" anything; we just suggest. If you like toast, by all means have it. If you don't like it, don't. Toasted or untoasted, the calorie count of bread (or rolls) is about the same.

"Whole-wheat bread" appears on your menus more frequently than other breads. Any reason?

Provided the bread is enriched, you can choose any non-whole-grain bread instead. Enriched means adding vitamins and minerals that are lost in processing. However, even enriched products may be low in some vitamins and trace minerals that are partially removed from the whole grain in the milling process. For this reason, it's a good idea to include some whole-grain products—such as whole-wheat bread—in your menus. Whole-wheat bread also contributes more fiber than non-whole-grain bread.

Should pasta and breakfast cereals be enriched?

Yes, for the same reason bread is enriched (see previous question). Unless, of course, they're made from the whole grain, like whole-wheat macaroni or shredded wheat. Most breakfast cereals are "fortified" (the word means "strengthened," and is equivalent to "enriched") at nutrient levels higher than those occurring in natural whole grains. In fact, some fortified cereals include vitamins not found in natural cereals (vitamins A, B-12, C and D). But some other vitamins and trace minerals that have been processed out may not have been reprocessed in; so, play it safe and include some whole-grain pasta and breakfast cereals in your menus. Many people find them delicious.

Why "unsweetened" breakfast cereals?

Sugar offers nothing nutritionally except calories (energy). That's why it's called an "empty-calorie" food. When sugar makes up a substantial share of your calories, it's likely to replace other foods that offer vitamins, minerals and proteins as well as energy. Many breakfast cereals contain 40 to 60 percent sugar by weight. Because sugar is well liked, it's easy to eat more of a sugar product than you realize—and the calories mount up surprisingly fast. Unsweetened cereals are naturally delicious.

Cereals seem to dominate your breakfast menus. Any special reason?

If you customarily build your breakfast around cereal, you start the day off consuming less fat, saturated fat, cholesterol, sodium and calories than you would on "bacon-and-egg-type" breakfast fare. Cereal grains are an excellent source of dietary fiber as well. But cereal-based breakfasts are not mandatory. Your first meal of the day can feature meat, fish, fowl, fruit, vegetables or anything that pleases you.

Why aren't granolas included on your menus?

Some commercial granolas contain up to five times more fat than most breakfast cereals; and much of the fat, which is derived from hydrogenated vegetable oils and coconut oil, is saturated. On the other hand, most granolas are high in protein. On page 181, you'll find a recipe for a granola-type cereal. If you choose to start your day with granola, eat fewer fat calories for the rest of the day.

I like to munch on dry shredded wheat biscuits. Anything wrong with that?

Nothing. Lots of people do. But drink your milk anyway. There's not much calcium in cereals, and milk is the best dietary source of this essential mineral. There may be a shortage of calcium in some average American diets.

What's better for me—"instant" hot cereals or the regular kind that I have to cook for up to ten minutes?

There's not much difference between the two nutritionally, with one exception. "Instant" or "quick" cereals are usually considerably higher in sodium. One "regular" oatmeal contains less than ten milligrams of sodium per serving; the "instant" equivalent, four hundred.

How much sodium do some popular brands of breakfast cereal contain?

In the less-than-ten-milligrams-a-serving class, you'll find shredded wheat, Puffed Wheat, Puffed Rice, Wheatena, Maltex, Regular Quaker Oatmeal, and Cream of Wheat. In the less-than-two-hundred-milligrams-a-serving class, there are Grape Nuts, Product 19, Most, All-Bran, and Nutri-Grain. Most other breakfast cereals contain more than two hundred milligrams, with some in the three hundred to four hundred milligrams range. Read the nutritional information on labels.

What's your advice on the choice of salad dressings?

The choice is, of course, yours. But you'll find some facts on the following page that will help you come to a decision.

"You can brown-paper-bag this one." Really? *You tell* me *how I'm going to carry a tossed salad with dressing in a paper bag.*

It's easy as 1-2-3.

1. For the salad. Fill a wide-mouth Thermos with cold water. Let stand for five minutes. Pour out the water. Fill with salad greens. Close Thermos.

2. For the dressing, cut down a bag-sealer bag to size. Insert dressing. Seal.

3. Pack brown paper bag with filled Thermos and bag-sealer bag.

COMPOSITION OF SELECTED SALAD DRESSINGS[1]

	In 1 Tablespoon		
Salad Dressing	Calories	Fat[2]	Sodium[3]
Blue and Roquefort			
Regular	76	7.8	164
Low-fat	3-12	.2-.9	170-177
French			
Regular	66	6.2	219
Low-fat	15	.7	126
Italian			
Regular	83	9.0	314
Low-fat	8	.7	118
Mayonnaise			
Regular	101	11.2	84
Mayonnaise-type	65	6.3	88
Mayonnaise-type, dietary	22	2.0	19
Russian	74	7.6	130
Thousand Island			
Regular	80	8.0	112
Dietary	27	2.1	105

[1] Information derived from *Agriculture Handbook No. 456*, published by the Agricultural Research Service, U.S. Department of Agriculture.

[2] In grams

[3] In milligrams

You may need to purchase a wide-mouth Thermos and a bag sealer plus a supply of bag-sealer bags, but the price is right. You may like to make one additional small purchase— an insulated lunch box. It will do wonders for your fruits, raw vegetables and sandwiches. Buying lunch-carrying equipment is a sound investment. You'll save on the cost of eat-out lunches, and you'll help avoid spoilage.

For information on "Safe Brown-Bag Lunches," write for the pamphlet of that title to FSIS Information, U.S. Department of Agriculture, Washington, D.C. 20250. It's free.

I just won't *carry my lunch. What's your answer to that?*

Eat out. Try to match the suggested lunch menus (Chapters 2 and 3) or make substitutions (pages 94–107), or make up your own menus (Chapter 6).

There are some lunches on your menus that simply can't be brown-paper-bagged or eaten out. I can't eat my lunches at home. What am I to do?

We've emphasized that you don't have to follow our menus. Make up lunch menus that you *can* eat out (Chapter 6).

May I drink mineral water instead of tap water?

Yes. But some mineral waters have laxative effects. Why not ask your doctor about the mineral waters you have in mind?

May I substitute herb teas for tea?

Jane E. Brody warns that teas made of any of the following ingredients are to be avoided as possibly hazardous to your health: sassafras bark, senna, burdock, juniper berries, shave grass (horsetail), dock, aloe, catnip, hydrangea, lobelia, jimson weed, wormwood, poke, licorice (in large amounts), ginseng, mandrake, snakeroot, St.-John's-wort, yohimbé, periwinkle, thorn apple, as well as the pits, bark and leaves of apricot, bitter almond, casava beans, cherry, chokecherry, peach, pear, apple and plum. If you have a ragweed or similar allergy, stay away from the flower heads of yarrow, marigold, chamomile and goldenrod. On the other hand, most other herbal teas are harmless. It would be wise to check with your doctor before adding herbal teas to your menu.

Your recipes give no specific quantities for coffee or tea. Why?

The government nutritionists leave the choice of the amount of these beverages up to you, with the caution: moderation in all things. Although excess caffeine (the basic stimulant in coffee and tea) can affect your mental and physical health adversely, most Americans can drink up to two cups of coffee or four cups of tea a day without any harm. However, caffeine tolerance varies from person to person; so you should think about setting your own caffeine limit by consulting with your doctor. Remember, there's also caffeine in many soft drinks, cocoa and chocolate.

Is it safe to use sugar substitutes in my coffee or tea?

Saccharin, a noncaloric sweetener, is a suspected carcinogen. The Food and Drug Administration, however, permits its sale, and both the American Diabetic Association and the American Dietetic Association allow its use in limited quantities for diabetics. Saccharin products are marketed as Sucaryl Sodium, Sweets and Sweet 'n Low. Caloric sweeteners such as fructose, xylitol and sorbitol are sugars roughly equivalent calorically to table sugar (sucrose). New sugar substitutes are likely to be introduced on the market. Before using them, or any other sugar substitute, check with your doctor.

5

The Maintenance Diets for Women and Men

STAYING AT YOUR ideal weight healthfully involves menus based on The Federal Dietary Guidelines. They are the same kind of menus that helped you reduce. You can make the transition from a reducing diet to a maintenance diet simply by continuing to practice the principles of the new nutrition, and raising the number of calories you consume daily.

Here are two versions of maintenance diets prepared by the Department of Agriculture nutritionists.* They reflect the amounts of food that women and men say they eat, on the average, as reported in surveys. They also represent (as do the reducing diets) the foods most Americans commonly eat, and the way those foods are usually prepared. The 1,600-calorie maintenance diet is intended for most women and small-frame men. The 2,400-calorie diet is intended for most men and large-frame women.

The calorie level in these menus is not necessarily right for you, since we all vary greatly in our need for calories. If

---

*The menus in this chapter appear in *Ideas for Better Eating,* published by the Science and Education Administration/Human Nutrition, U. S. Department of Agriculture.

you're physically active or heavier than the average American man or woman, you may need more calories than the amounts in these menus; if you're not very active and weigh less than the average American man or woman, you may need fewer calories. Experiment with eating less or more than the amounts called for in these menus until you arrive at just the right amount of food to keep your weight steady. Check on your weight weekly, and make your adjustments depending on whether you've gained or lost on the previous week's menus.

Like the reducing menus, the maintenance menus can be followed as-is, or they can be modified to suit your own preferences (see Chapter 6). They are, in essence, blueprints for a lifetime of healthful, stay-slim and enjoyable eating.

THE MAINTENANCE DIET FOR MOST WOMEN (AND SMALL-FRAME MEN)

Day 1

BREAKFAST
- ¾ cup orange juice, fresh or frozen
- 2 slices banana-nut bread (1)
- ½ cup skim milk (fortified)
- water, tea or coffee

LUNCH
(You can brown-paper-bag this one)
- 1 tuna-salad sandwich, consisting of:
  - • 2 ounces canned tuna, packed in water
  - • 1 tablespoon chopped celery
  - • 1 teaspoon chopped onion
  - • 2 teaspoons mayonnaise
  - • 2 slices whole-wheat bread
- 1 medium pear, fresh
- 1 cup skim milk, fortified

DINNER
- 4 ounces pot roast, chuck, lean only
- ¾ cup mashed potatoes
- ½ cup green beans, fresh or frozen
- 1 cup spinach salad, with
- 1 tablespoon Italian dressing
- 1 slice Italian bread, enriched, with
- 1 teaspoon margarine, soft
- ½ cup orange-pineapple cup (2)
- water, tea or coffee

(1) See recipe, page 180.
(2) See recipe, page 169.

SNACKS
- ¼ cup chili bean dip (3)
- 1 cup raw vegetable sticks: carrot, celery and green pepper sticks

  water, tea or coffee

(3) See recipe, page 222.

Day 2

BREAKFAST
- ½ cup strawberries, fresh or frozen, unsweetened
- 2 biscuits shredded wheat, with
- ½ medium sliced banana
- 1 cup low-fat milk (2 percent), fortified

  water, tea or coffee

LUNCH
- 1 hamburger, consisting of:
  - 2 ounces ground beef
  - enriched bun
- ½ cup coleslaw, with mayonnaise-type salad dressing
- 1 small serving french fries
- 8 ounces juice or alternate (1)

DINNER
- 1 serving chicken cacciatore (2)
- ½ cup spaghetti, enriched
- ½ cup zucchini, cooked, fresh

(1) See list of alternates, page 106.
(2) See recipe, page 221.

1½ cups mixed green salad: iceberg lettuce, spinach,
     green onions, cucumbers, with
1   tablespoon Italian dressing
1   slice Italian bread, enriched, with
1   teaspoon margarine, soft

SNACKS
½ cup low-fat milk (2 percent), fortified
1 medium tangerine

Day 3

BREAKFAST
¾ cup orange juice, fresh or frozen
1 bagel
1 tablespoon cream cheese
1 cup skim milk, fortified
   water, tea or coffee

LUNCH
(You can brown-paper-bag this one)
1 sliced chicken sandwich, consisting of:
    • 2 ounces sliced chicken
    • 1 leaf lettuce
    • 2 teaspoons mayonnaise-type salad dressing
    • 2 slices whole-wheat bread
1 serving bean salad (1)
   water, tea or coffee

DINNER
1 serving vegetable chowder (2)

(1) See recipe, page 218.
(2) See recipe, page 175.

1   serving spicy baked fish (3)
½   cup broccoli spears, fresh or frozen
½   cup brown rice
1½ cups mixed green salad: iceberg lettuce, spinach,
      green onions, cucumbers, with
1   tablespoon French dressing
½   cup grapes, seedless
    water, tea or coffee

SNACK
1   serving gingerbread (4)

(3) See recipe, page 222.
(4) See recipe, page 191.

Day 4

BREAKFAST
¼   medium cantaloupe
1   large egg, soft cooked
1   average corn muffin
½   cup low-fat milk (1 percent), fortified
    water, tea or coffee

LUNCH
1   ham and cheese sandwich, consisting of:
    • 1 ounce lean ham
    • 1 ounce natural Swiss cheese
    • 2 slices rye bread
    • 2 teaspoons mayonnaise-type salad dressing
    • lettuce
1¼ cups tossed salad: lettuce, tomato, carrots, green
      onions, with
1   tablespoon Italian dressing
1   medium orange
    water, tea or coffee

DINNER

1   serving flounder Florentine (1)
1   medium baked potato, with
2   tablespoons sour cream
½   cup green peas, frozen
1   small whole-wheat roll
1   teaspoon margarine, soft
4   ounces vanilla yogurt, low-fat, mixed with
½   cup strawberries, fresh or frozen, unsweetened
     water, tea or coffee

SNACK

1   whole English muffin, enriched, with
1   tablespoon marmalade

(1) See recipe, page 219.

Day 5

BREAKFAST

½   medium grapefruit, fresh
2   slices whole-wheat toast
1   teaspoon margarine, soft
1   cup skim milk, fortified
     water, tea or coffee

LUNCH

(You can brown-paper-bag this one)

6   ounces tomato juice, canned
1   serving luncheon salad, consisting of:
     • 1½ cups mixed greens
     • 1½ ounces natural Swiss cheese
     • 1 tablespoon French dressing

1   serving corn bread (1)
1   small peach, fresh
     water, tea or coffee

DINNER

4   ounces broiled ground beef, lean
½   cup corn, fresh or frozen
½   cup green beans, fresh or frozen
1   serving baked apple, with
2   teaspoons brown sugar
     water, tea or coffee

SNACK

8   ounces juice or alternate (2)

(1) See recipe, page 189.
(2) See list of alternates, page 106.

Day 6

BREAKFAST

¾   cup orange juice, fresh or frozen
2   whole-wheat pancakes (1)
½   serving blueberry sauce (2)
1   cup low-fat milk (1 percent), fortified
     water, tea or coffee

LUNCH

1   beef taco (3)
¾   cup fresh fruit cup: oranges, apples, bananas
½   cup low-fat milk (1 percent), fortified

(1) See recipe, page 182.
(2) See recipe, page 172.
(3) See recipe, page 208.

DINNER

4   ounces roast loin of pork, lean only
1   small sweet potato, baked
½   cup collard greens, fresh or frozen
1¼ cups tossed salad: lettuce, tomato, green onions, carrots, with
1   tablespoon Italian salad dressing
1   biscuit, enriched, with
1   teaspoon margarine, soft
     water, tea or coffee

SNACKS

4   squares graham crackers
8   ounces juice or alternate (4)

(4) See list of alternates, page 106.

Day 7

BREAKFAST

½   cup pineapple chunks, packed in own juice
½   cup oatmeal, with cinnamon and
1   teaspoon brown sugar
½   cup low-fat milk (1 percent), fortified
     water, tea or coffee

LUNCH

1   serving split-pea soup (1)
1   serving chicken salad stuffed tomato, consisting of:
     • 2 ounces cooked, chopped chicken
     • 1 tablespoon chopped celery
     • 1 teaspoon chopped onion

(1) See recipe, page 202.

- 2 teaspoons mayonnaise
- medium tomato

3   rye crackers
     water, tea or coffee

DINNER

1   serving beef with Chinese-style vegetables (2)
½   cup rice, white, enriched
1   serving apple crisp (3)

SNACKS

2   slices banana-nut bread (4)
1   cup low-fat (1 percent) milk, fortified
1   medium orange

(2) See recipe, page 220.
(3) See recipe, page 173.
(4) See recipe, page 180.

THE MAINTENANCE DIET FOR MOST MEN (AND LARGE-FRAME WOMEN)

Day 1

BREAKFAST

¾ cup orange juice, fresh or frozen
1 large egg, soft cooked
2 slices banana-nut bread (1)
1 cup skim milk, fortified
  water, tea or coffee

LUNCH

(You can brown-paper-bag this one)

1 tuna salad sandwich, consisting of:
  • 2 ounces tuna, packed in water
  • 1 tablespoon chopped celery
  • 1 teaspoon chopped onion
  • 2 teaspoons mayonnaise
  • 2 slices whole-wheat bread
1 medium pear, fresh
1 cup skim milk, fortified

DINNER

4 ounces pot roast, chuck, lean only
¾ cup mashed potatoes
½ cup green beans, fresh or frozen
1 cup spinach salad, with
1 tablespoon Italian dressing
2 slices Italian bread, enriched, with
1 tablespoon margarine, soft
1 cup orange-pineapple cup (2)
  water, tea or coffee

(1) See recipe, page 180.
(2) See recipe, page 169.

SNACKS

½ cup chili bean dip (3)

1 cup raw vegetable sticks: carrot, celery and green
    pepper sticks

5 to 6 average whole-wheat crackers

12 ounces juice or alternate (4)
    water, tea or coffee

(3) See recipe, page 222.
(4) See list of alternates, page 106.

Day 2

BREAKFAST

½ cup strawberries, fresh or frozen, unsweetened

2 biscuits shredded wheat, with

½ medium sliced banana

1 tablespoon sugar

1 cup low-fat milk (2 percent), fortified
    water, tea or coffee

LUNCH

1 hamburger/cheeseburger, consisting of:
    • 3 ounces ground beef
    • ¾ ounce processed American cheese
    • 1 enriched bun

½ cup coleslaw, with mayonnaise-type salad dressing

1 large serving french fries

8 ounces juice or alternate (1)

(1) See list of alternates, page 106.

DINNER

1   serving chicken cacciatore (2)
1   cup spaghetti, enriched
½   cup zucchini, cooked fresh
1½ cups mixed green salad: iceberg lettuce, spinach,
       green onions, cucumbers, with
1   tablespoon Italian dressing
2   slices Italian bread, enriched, with
2   teaspoons margarine, soft
1   medium pear, fresh
1   cup pineapple juice, unsweetened

SNACKS

2   squares graham crackers
½   cup low-fat milk (2 percent), fortified
1   medium tangerine

(2) See recipe, page 221.

Day 3

BREAKFAST

¾   cup orange juice, fresh or frozen
1   large scrambled egg
1   bagel, with
2   tablespoons cream cheese, and
1   tablespoon jam
1   cup skim milk, fortified
     water, tea or coffee

LUNCH

(You can brown-paper-bag this one)

2   sliced chicken sandwiches, consisting of:
     • 3 ounces sliced chicken
     • 2 leaves lettuce
     • 3 teaspoons mayonnaise-type salad dressing
     • 4 slices whole-wheat bread

1 serving bean salad (1)
1 medium apple, fresh
water, tea or coffee

DINNER

1 serving vegetable chowder (2)
1½ servings spicy baked fish (3)
½ cup broccoli spears, fresh or frozen
½ cup brown rice
1½ cups mixed green salad: iceberg lettuce, spinach,
green onions, cucumbers, with
1 tablespoon French dressing
1 cup grapes, seedless
water, tea or coffee

SNACKS

1 serving gingerbread (4)
1 medium pear, fresh

(1) See recipe, page 218.
(2) See recipe, page 175.
(3) See recipe, page 222.
(4) See recipe, page 191.

Day 4

BREAKFAST

¼ medium cantaloupe
2 average corn muffins, with
2 teaspoons margarine, soft, and
2 teaspoons jelly
1 cup low-fat milk (1 percent), fortified
water, tea or coffee

LUNCH

  1   large pork chop, lean only
  ½   cup black-eyed peas
  ½   cup rice, enriched
  1   large hard roll, enriched, with
  1   teaspoon margarine, soft
  ½   cup sliced peaches, canned in syrup
  ¾   cup apple cider

DINNER

  1   serving flounder florentine (1)
  1   medium baked potato, with
  2   tablespoons sour cream
  ½   cup green peas, frozen
  1   small whole-wheat roll
  1   teaspoon margarine, soft
  8   ounces vanilla yogurt, low-fat, mixed with
  ½   cup strawberries, fresh or frozen, unsweetened
       water, tea or coffee

SNACKS

  1   whole English muffin, enriched, with
  2   teaspoons margarine, soft, and
  1   tablespoon marmalade

(1) See recipe, page 219.

Day 5

BREAKFAST

  ½   medium grapefruit, fresh
  2   slices whole-wheat toast, with
  1   teaspoon margarine, soft and
  1   tablespoon jelly

1   cup skim milk, fortified
    water, tea or coffee

LUNCH
(You can brown-paper-bag this one)
6   ounces tomato juice, canned
1   serving luncheon salad, consisting of:
    • 2 ounces turkey
    • 1 ounce ham
    • 1½ cups mixed greens
    • 1½ ounces natural Swiss cheese
    • 1½ tablespoons French dressing
1   serving corn bread (1)
2   small peaches, fresh
    water, tea or coffee

DINNER
4   ounces broiled ground beef, lean
1   cup corn, fresh or frozen
½   cup green beans, fresh or frozen
2   rye rolls, with
1   teaspoon margarine, soft
1   serving baked apple, with
2   teaspoons brown sugar
    water, tea or coffee

SNACKS
1   peanut butter sandwich, consisting of:
    • 2 slices whole-wheat bread
    • 2 tablespoons peanut butter
    • 2 teaspoons jelly
8   ounces juice or alternate (2)

(1) See recipe, page 189.
(2) See list of alternates, page 106.

Day 6

BREAKFAST

¾ cup orange juice, fresh or frozen
3 whole-wheat pancakes (1), with
1 serving blueberry sauce (2)
1 cup low-fat milk, (1 percent), fortified
2 teaspoons margarine, soft
   water, tea or coffee

LUNCH

2 beef tacos (3)
¾ cup fresh fruit cup: oranges, apples, bananas
1 cup low-fat milk (1 percent), fortified

DINNER

4 ounces roast loin of pork, lean only
1 medium sweet potato, baked
½ cup collard greens, fresh or frozen
1¼ cups tossed salad: lettuce, tomato, green onions,
    carrots, with
1 tablespoon Italian salad dressing
2 biscuits, enriched, with
1 tablespoon honey, and
2 teaspoons margarine, soft
   water, tea or coffee

SNACKS

4 squares graham crackers
12 ounces juice or alternate (4)
1 medium apple, fresh

(1) See recipe, page 182.
(2) See recipe, page 172.
(3) See recipe, page 208.
(4) See list of alternates, page 106.

Day 7

BREAKFAST
- ¾ cup pineapple chunks, packed in own juice
- 1 cup oatmeal with cinnamon, and
- 3 tablespoons raisins, and
- 2 teaspoons brown sugar
- 1 cup low-fat milk (1 percent), fortified
water, tea or coffee

LUNCH
- 1 serving split-pea soup (1)
- 1 serving chicken salad stuffed tomato, consisting of:
  - 2 ounces cooked, chopped chicken
  - 1 tablespoon chopped celery
  - 1 teaspoon chopped onion
  - 2 teaspoons mayonnaise
  - 1 medium tomato
- 6 rye crackers, with
- 2 teaspoons margarine, soft
- ¾ cup lemon sherbet
water, tea or coffee

DINNER
- 1½ servings beef with Chinese-style vegetables (2)
- ¾ cup rice, white, enriched
- 1 serving apple crisp (3)

SNACKS
- 2 slices banana-nut bread (4)
- 1 cup low-fat milk (1 percent), fortified
- 1 medium orange

(1) See recipe, page 202.
(2) See recipe, page 220.
(3) See recipe, page 173.
(4) See recipe, page 180.

6

How to Make Up Your Own Maintenance and Reducing Menus

THE EASIEST WAY is to use the menus in this book as guides. They show you how to put together nutritious meals and snacks. They are examples, not commandments. Pick the ones that suit your own eating habits best, then adapt them to your needs by making substitutions liberally from the four basic food groups, and cautiously from the fifth. The five food groups are:

1. Fruit-Vegetable
2. Bread-Cereal
3. Milk-Cheese
4. Meat-Poultry-Fish-Beans
5. Fats-Sweets-Alcohol

Choices are arranged in two columns under each of the five group headings. The first column is titled *Choices in Our Menus*, and lists the items with which Department of Agriculture nutritionists created their menus in this book. The second column is titled *Other Choices*, and lists foods that, while not exactly equivalent in nutrient content to the items in the first column, come close enough. In creating your own menus, you can use items from either column, or from both.* For alternates to juices, see page 106.

When you make substitutions, choose foods from the same food groups as the ones in the menu. Be varied in your choices. And remember these

FOUR BASIC RULES
FOR MAKING UP YOUR OWN MENUS

1. Eat a variety of foods in moderation, and avoid imbalanced or excessive consumption.

2. Get enough of the basic foods and nutrients without overdoing the calories.

3. Cut back on those ingredients or foods that you may eat too much of—fats and oils, salt and sugar.

4. Select at least four servings a day from each of the Fruit-Vegetable and Bread-Cereal groups, and at least two servings a day from each of the Milk-Cheese and the Meat-Poultry-Fish-Beans groups.

1. CHOICES IN THE FRUIT-VEGETABLE GROUP

Fruit

Make substitutions by "servings." Count as a serving in the fruit group: a whole piece of fruit (average size), a melon wedge, 6 ounces of juice, ½ cup berries or ½ cup of sliced or cooked fruit.

*The lists of choices in this chapter appear in *Ideas for Better Eating*, published by the Science and Education Administration/Human Nutrition, U.S. Department of Agriculture.

Choices in the menus
    Apples
    Apple cider
    Apple crisp
      (see recipe, page 173)
    Baked apple
    Bananas
    Cantaloupes
    Fruit cup
    Grapefruit
    Grapes
    Oranges
    Orange juice
    Orange-pineapple cup
      (see recipe, page 169)
    Peaches, fresh and canned
    Pears
    Pineapple, canned in own juice
    Raisins
    Strawberries
    Tangerines
    Tomatoes and tomato juice

Other Choices
    Applesauce
    Apricots
    Blueberries and other berries
    Cherries
    Figs
    Honeydew melon
    Lemons
    Mangoes
    Nectarines
    Papayas
    Plums

Prunes
Watermelon
Other fruit and fruit juices

Vegetables

Make substitutions by "servings." Count as a serving in the vegetable group: a typical serving, a ½ cup, a wedge of lettuce, a small salad, or 1 medium potato.

There are three types of vegetables to include in your menus: dark-green vegetables, starchy vegetables, and other vegetables. Each type makes a somewhat different contribution to your diet. It is wise to eat one starchy vegetable or bean dish daily; and dark-green vegetables should show up often.

1. DARK-GREEN VEGETABLES

Choices in the menus
    Broccoli
    Collard greens
    Spinach (cooked or raw)

Other Choices
    Chicory
    Endive
    Escarole
    Greens, including:
        Beet
        Chard
        Dandelion
        Kale
        Mustard

Turnip
Romaine lettuce
Watercress

2. STARCHY VEGETABLES

Choices in the menus
Black-eyed peas
Chili bean dip
(see recipe, page 222)
Corn
Green peas
Bean salad
(see recipe, page 218)
Potatoes, including:
Baked
French fried
Mashed
Split-pea soup
(see recipe, page 202)
Sweet potatoes

Other Choices
Chickpeas or garbanzos
Lentils
Lima beans
Navy beans
Parsnips
Plantains
Rutabaga
Yams
Other types of dried
beans and peas

3. OTHER VEGETABLES

Choices in the menus
Carrots
Celery
Coleslaw (cabbage)
Cucumbers
Green beans
Green peppers
Lettuce (iceberg, bibb)
Onions (mature and green)
Tomatoes and tomato juice
Vegetables in main-dish recipes
Vegetables in vegetable chowder
(see recipe, page 175)
Zucchini

Other Choices
Artichokes
Asparagus
Bean and alfalfa sprouts
Beets
Brussels sprouts
Cauliflower
Chinese cabbage
Eggplant
Mushrooms
Okra
Pumpkin
Radishes
Turnips
Vegetable juices
Winter squash
Yellow squash
Other vegetables

2. CHOICES IN THE BREAD-CEREAL GROUP

This group includes all grain products, either whole or enriched. Make substitutions by "servings." Count as a serving in this group: 1 slice bread; ½ to ¾ cup cooked cereal, cornmeal, grits, macaroni, noodles, rice or spaghetti; and 1 ounce ready-to-eat cereal.

Choices in the menus
    Bagel
    Banana-nut bread
        (see recipe, page 180)
    Biscuits
    Brown rice
    Corn bread
        (see recipe, page 189)
    Corn muffins
    English muffins
    Gingerbread
        (see recipe, page 191)
    Graham crackers
    Hamburger bun
    Italian bread
    Oatmeal
    Ready-to-eat cereal (Shredded Wheat)
    Rice
    Rye bread
    Rye crackers
    Rye rolls
    Spaghetti
    Taco shells
    Wheat crackers
    Whole-wheat bread

Whole-wheat pancakes
(see recipe, page 182)
Whole-wheat rolls

Other Choices
Barley
Buckwheat groats
Bulgur
Cornmeal
Grits
Muffins
Noodles, macaroni
Popcorn
Pumpernickel bread
Waffles
White bread
Wild rice
Other breads and cereals

Caution: Before making your choice, check the ingredient label or the recipe for added salt, sugar, or fat. Quick breads, such as muffins, biscuits and corn bread, have more fat than most yeast breads. Think about how much fat you add in cooking or at the table.

3. CHOICES IN THE MILK-CHEESE GROUP

This group includes milk in any form. Make substitutions by "servings." Count as a serving in this group: 1 cup milk, 1 cup yogurt, 1⅓ ounces Cheddar or Swiss cheese, 2 ounces processed cheese food, 1½ cups ice cream or ice milk, or 2 cups cottage cheese.

When preparing your menus, you can trade off some members of this group for other members, sometimes plus certain quantities of sugar and/or fat. The trade-offs are approximately equal in calories, calcium, protein, fat and total carbohydrate content.

MILK PRODUCTS TRADE-OFFS

1 cup whole milk	for	1 cup skim milk plus 2 teaspoons fat
1 cup 2 percent low-fat milk	for	1 cup skim milk plus 2 teaspoons fat
1½ ounces natural cheese	for	1 cup whole milk plus 1 teaspoon fat
8 ounces plain low-fat yogurt	for	1 cup 2 percent low-fat milk
1 cup low-fat (2 percent) chocolate milk	for	1 cup 2 percent low-fat milk plus 3 teaspoons sugar
8 ounces low-fat vanilla yogurt	for	1 cup 2 percent low-fat milk plus 4 teaspoons sugar
8 ounces low-fat fruit yogurt	for	1 cup 2 percent low-fat milk plus 7 teaspoons sugar
½ cup ice cream	for	⅓ cup skim milk plus 2 teaspoons fat plus 3 teaspoons sugar
½ cup ice milk	for	⅓ cup skim milk plus 4 teaspoons sugar

Choices in the menu
　　American cheese
　　Low-fat milk (1 percent and 2 percent)
　　Milk in vegetable chowder
　　　(see recipe, page 175)
　　Skim milk
　　Swiss cheese
　　Vanilla low-fat yogurt
　　Whole milk

*Other Choices**
Buttermilk
Chocolate milk
Cottage cheese
Low-fat yogurt, plain
Milk custards
Milk puddings
Other cheeses

Caution: Cottage cheese contains considerably less calcium than other cheeses. One-half cup of cottage cheese contains only as much calcium as is found in one-quarter cup of milk, while providing considerably more calories and sodium.

4. CHOICES IN THE MEAT-POULTRY-FISH-BEANS GROUP

Eggs, nuts, peanut butter, seeds, peas and lentils are also included in this group. Make substitutions by "servings." Count a serving in this group as: 2 to 3 ounces of lean, boneless cooked meat, poultry or fish; 2 eggs; 1 to 1½ cups cooked dry beans, peas, lentils or soybeans; 4 tablespoons peanut butter; or ½ to 1 cup nuts, sesame or sunflower seeds.

For 2 ounces of lean meat, fish, or poultry plus 2 slices of whole-wheat bread, you can trade off 1 cup of cooked dry beans or peas plus 1 teaspoon fat.

Choices in the menus
Spicy baked fish
(see recipe, page 222)

*For the calorie, fat and sodium content of popular cheeses, see page 67.

Beef pot roast
Beef tacos
    (see recipe, page 208)
Beef with Chinese-style vegetables
    (see recipe, page 220)
Chicken
Chicken cacciatore
    (see recipe, page 221)
Eggs, scrambled and soft cooked
Eggs in recipes
Flounder Florentine
    (see recipe, page 219)
Ground beef (lean)
Ham
Pork chops
Pork loin roast
Tuna fish
Turkey

Other Choices
Beef, macaroni and tomato casserole
Beef stew
Beef, other lean cuts
Chili
Lamb chop or roast (lean)
Lamb stew
Meat loaf
Pork, other lean cuts
Shellfish and other fish
Veal

5. CHOICES IN THE FATS-SWEETS-ALCOHOL GROUP

This group includes foods like butter, margarine, mayonnaise and other salad dressings, and other fats and oils; candy, sugar, jams, jellies, syrups, sweet toppings and other sweets; soft drinks and other highly sugared beverages; and alcoholic beverages such as wine, beer and hard liquor. Also included are refined but unenriched breads, pastries and flour products. Some of these foods are used as ingredients in prepared foods or are added to other foods at the table. Others are just "extras."

No serving sizes are defined, because a basic number of servings is not suggested for this group.

Fats and Oils

Animal fats are higher in saturated fat than are most vegetable oils. The exceptions are coconut and palm oil. These vegetable oils are highly saturated. It is not a good idea to use highly saturated fats exclusively. Soft (tub) margarine is a good choice as a spread for bread and vegetables. It is made from liquid vegetable oils that have been only partially hardened (hydrogenated). Remember to use fats and oils with moderation.

Choices in the menus
    Cream cheese
    French and Italian salad dressing
    Margarine (soft)
    Mayonnaise
    Mayonnaise-type salad dressing
    Oil (in recipes)
    Sour cream

Other Choices
   Bacon
   Butter
   Cream
   Half-and-half
   Nondairy creamers
   Margarine (hard)
   Other types of salad dressing

Sugar and Sweets

Sugars and sweets are listed in the menus. They are also found in prepared foods like salad dressings, peanut butter, vanilla yogurt, lemon sherbet and quick breads. The amount of sugar we include in the recipes is lower than you will find in many cookbooks.

Calorie levels are somewhat similar for the sugars and sweeteners listed below. They can be substituted, teaspoon for teaspoon. It is hard to tell how much sugar has been added to foods like peanut butter, catsup or ready-to-eat cereal. Read the label. Ingredients are listed in order of predominance. If sugar or some other caloric sweetener comes first, you know there is more sugar than anything else. It is a great deal easier to control the amount of sugar in your food if you add it yourself. Honey and brown sugar are used for their flavor and color. They have no other special value.

Caution: Words used on labels to describe sugar and caloric sweeteners include sugar, sucrose, dextrose, fructose, corn syrups, corn sweeteners, natural sweeteners, honey and invert sugar.

Choices in the menus
   Blueberry sauce
      (see recipe, page 172)

Honey
Jam
Jelly
Marmalade
Sugar (white and brown)
Syrup on peaches

Other Choices
Corn syrup
Maple syrup
Molasses
Sugar syrup

Alcohol

Not recommended on weight-reduction menus. On maintenance menus, use cautiously, and compensate for the extra calories by decreasing some portions of your other foods. After all, alcohol with its seven calories per gram, as opposed to four calories from carbohydrates and proteins, and nine from fats, can add an appreciable caloric load to your diet.

ALTERNATES TO JUICES

An 8-ounce glass of juice contributes about 110 calories. The following alternates contribute about the same number of calories:

8   ounces fruit punch
8   ounces soft drink
½   cup sherbet (also contains some fat)
1   popsicle
¾   cup sweetened gelatin

2   average cookies (also contain some fat)
2   tablespoons sugar, jam, jelly, honey, syrup
1   ounce candy (some contain fat)
8   ounces beer
4   ounces table wine
1½ ounces whiskey

We're not advocating the use of alcoholic beverages. We are only indicating where they fit if you choose to use them.

HOW TO ADJUST YOUR MAINTENANCE DIET TO YOUR CALORIC NEEDS

How do you know whether a 1,600-calorie-a-day diet or 2,400-calorie-a-day diet will keep your weight steady? Before going on either of these maintenance diets, weigh yourself. Then, a week later at about the same time of day, weigh yourself again. If you lost weight, you need more calories; if you gained weight, you need fewer calories.

To adjust your maintenance diet to cut your caloric intake, follow these

SEVEN NUTRITIONAL GUIDELINES TO PERMANENT SLIMNESS

1. Cut down on high-fat foods, such as margarine, butter, highly marbled or fatty meats and fried foods. Salad dressings, cream sauces, gravies and many whipped dessert toppings are also high in fat.
2. Cut down on sugary foods, such as candies; soft drinks and other sugar-sweetened beverages such as ades and

punches; jelly, jam, syrups, honey; fruit canned in heavy syrup; pies, cakes and pastries.

3. Cut down on or eliminate alcoholic drinks.

4. Cut down on portion sizes. Portions of some foods, such as meats, are hard to estimate. For example, a 3-ounce serving of cooked lean meat without bone is equivalent to a 3- by ⅝-inch hamburger patty.

5. Use whole milk or whole-milk products (most cheeses and ice cream) sparingly. Low-fat and skim-milk products, such as ice milk and skim-milk cheeses, provide fewer calories than their whole-milk counterparts.

6. Select cooking methods to help cut calories. Cook foods with little or no added fat and avoid deep-fat fried foods, which are high in calories because of the fat absorbed during cooking. For meat and poultry, trim off visible fat; either broil or roast on a rack. If braised or stewed, drain meat to remove fat. For fish, broil or bake. For vegetables, steam, bake, or broil; for an occasional change, stir-fry in a small amount of vegetable oil.

7. Be sure to count the nibbles and drinks enjoyed during social events and throughout the day as part of your day's calorie allotment.

To adjust your maintenance diet to increase your caloric intake, reverse the preceding guidelines.

CALORIE ADJUSTMENT CHART

If you need to increase your caloric intake, read from left to right. If you need to decrease your caloric intake, read from right to left. Calorie values are shown within parentheses.

FOR THE FRUIT-VEGETABLE GROUP

Low-Calorie Food	Medium-Calorie Version	High-Calorie Version
1 cup raw-vegetable salad with dressing (40)	¾ cup raw-vegetable salad with 1 tablespoon French dressing (95)	½ cup potato salad (125)
½ cup cooked cabbage (15)	½ cup coleslaw (60)	2 rolls stuffed cabbage (260)
1 medium baked potato (95)	⅔ cup mashed potatoes prepared with milk and butter (125)	½ cup hashed brown potatoes (170)
1 medium raw apple (80)	1 sweetened baked apple (160)	⅛ of 9-inch apple pie (300)
½ cup fresh citrus sections (40)	½ cup jellied citrus salad (120)	½ cup lemon pudding (145)
½ cup cooked green beans (15)	½ cup stir-fried green beans (35)	½ cup green bean and mushroom casserole (70)
½ cup diced fresh pineapple (40)	½ cup canned pineapple chunks in natural juice (70)	½ cup canned pineapple chunks in heavy syrup (95)

FOR THE BREAD-CEREAL GROUP

Low-Calorie Food	Medium-Calorie Version	High-Calorie Version
1 cup plain cornflakes (95)	1 cup sugar-coated cornflakes (155)	½ cup crunchy cereal (see recipe page 181) (280–290)
½ cup steamed or boiled rice (85)	½ cup fried rice without meat (185)	½ cup rice pudding (235)

Low-Calorie Food	Medium-Calorie Version	High-Calorie Version
1 slice of bread (55 to 70)	1 corn muffin (125)	1 Danish pastry (275)
½ cup cooked noodles (100)	6 cheese ravioli with sauce (175)	1 cup lasagna (345)

FOR THE MILK-CHEESE GROUP

Low-Calorie Food	Medium-Calorie Version	High-Calorie Version
½ cup (single dip) ice milk (95)	½ cup (single dip) ice cream (135)	1 cup vanilla milkshake (255)
1 oz Cheddar cheese (115)	1 cup cheese soufflé (260)	1 cup macaroni and cheese (430)
8 fl oz carton plain low-fat yogurt (145)	8 fl oz carton vanilla-flavored yogurt (195)	8 fl oz carton yogurt with fruit or 2 dips frozen yogurt (225 to 240)

FOR THE MEAT-POULTRY-FISH-BEAN GROUP

Low-Calorie Food	Medium-Calorie Version	High-Calorie Version
2 oz broiled chicken (95)	½ fried chicken breast (2¾ oz) or 2 drumsticks (2½ oz) (160–180)	8 oz individual chicken pot pie (505)
3 oz lean hamburger (without bun) (185)	3 oz regular hamburger (without bun) (235)	3½ oz cheeseburger (without bun) (320)
3 oz lean roast beef (205)	3 oz Swiss steak (315)	⅔ cup beef stroganoff over noodles (525)
2½ oz broiled cod with butter or margarine (120)	2½ oz fried, breaded ocean perch (160)	2½ oz baked stuffed fish (½ cup bread stuffing) (325)

Low-Calorie Food	Medium-Calorie Version	High-Calorie Version
½ cup boiled navy beans (95)	1 cup navy bean soup (170)	1 cup baked navy beans (310)
3 oz boiled shrimp (100)	3 oz fried, breaded shrimp (190)	½ cup shrimp Newburg (285)

FOR THE FATS-SWEETS-ALCOHOL GROUP

Low-Calorie Food	Medium-Calorie Version	High-Calorie Version
1 teaspoon sugar (15)	2 tablespoons pancake syrup (120)	12 fl oz cola (145)
12 fl oz light beer or 3½ fl oz dry wine (85 to 95)	12 fl oz regular beer or 3½ fl oz sweet wine (140 to 150)	Tom Collins—1 fl oz gin & 6 fl oz Tom Collins mix (195)
3 oz popsicle (70)	½ cup (single dip) sherbet (135)	1.2 oz milk-chocolate candy bar (175)

7

Eating Habits That Help Keep You Thin

THE FEDERAL DIETARY GUIDELINES advises you to eat slowly. When you follow this advice, what you're doing is acquiring a new eating habit—a thin eating habit.

Let's see how this new habit can help keep you thin.

Eating slowly. When enough of your food has entered the bloodstream, an appetite-regulating mechanism at the base of the brain signals enough's enough, and you come away from the table feeling satisfied. It takes a certain amount of time before that happens. Should you rush through your meal before that time, the enough's enough signal will not go off, you'll not feel satisfied and you'll eat more.

Here's an example. Let's say it takes thirty minutes before your enough's enough signal goes off (the time varies from individual to individual). But you're a fast eater and you finish your meal in fifteen minutes. You're still hungry and you continue eating. By the time your enough's enough signal goes off, you'll have consumed two meals.

By eating slowly, you cut down on the amount of food you eat.

But how do you learn to eat slowly?

112

Eating rapidly is a habit—an automatic act or behavior. You can change any habit by taking two steps. First, become aware of your habit. Then, follow a behavior-modification program. These two steps have been successful in helping people stop smoking, overcome depression, and reduce and stay reduced.

Here's how you can apply these two steps to change your "fat" fast-eating habit to a "thin" slow-eating habit.

How to become aware of your fast-eating habit:

• When you dine with thin people, observe how much faster you finish your meal than they do.

• Bring a mirror to the table and watch yourself eat.

• If you have a motion-picture camera or a video recorder, take pictures of yourself eating. You may not smile when you see yourself on candid camera.

• Ask people who will give you an honest answer, "Do you think I eat too fast?"

How to apply a behavior-modification program to change your fast-eating habit into a slow-eating habit:

• Chew, chew, chew. One expert suggests you chew each mouthful twenty times before swallowing. Try it. Count, 1 . . . 2 . . . 3 . . . to 20. Then swallow. After a while, you won't have to count. You'll be chewing your food properly—naturally.

• Concentrate on the flavor of the food. To do it, you have to hold your food in your mouth longer. Gourmets chew slowly until the last bit of flavor is extracted.

• Sip, don't gulp. You can swig down your juice in two swallows, or you can take twenty sips. Try for the twenty sips, and *really* taste what you're drinking for a change.

• *Look at* your food. *Do* you before you pitch in? Chances are you only give it a passing glance. Take the time to enjoy the appearance of what you're eating. It sets a leisurely pace for the entire meal.

• Eat with your knife, fork and spoon—never with your

hands. That applies when you eat *anything*—a sandwich, a slice of bread, a roll or a piece of fruit. Eating with utensils takes more time than eating with your fingers.

• Eat *small* pieces. It takes time to cut your food into small pieces, and it takes more time to eat many small pieces than it does to eat fewer big pieces.

• Bring your food to your mouth slowly. Count 1-2-3 from plate to mouth. You'll soon forget you ever shoveled it in at high speed. Your dining partners will appreciate the change to a more graceful you. You'll want to stay that way.

• Put only one kind of food in your mouth at a time. Not steak, potatoes and onions in one mouthful. But one mouthful of steak. One mouthful of potatoes. One mouthful of onions. That's three mouthfuls instead of one, and that takes three times longer to consume.

• Put down your utensils after they've delivered the food to your mouth. Finish chewing, then count to ten before you pick them up again.

• Don't eat continuously. Talk to your dinner partners instead (never with food in your mouth).

• Take time out between courses. Your next course will taste so much better that you'll rapidly make this a standard practice. Take the longest time out before your dessert. You'll be astonished by how much less you'll eat of that pie, ice cream, custard or other goodies.

OTHER THIN EATING HABITS YOU CAN ACQUIRE BY CHANGING YOUR BEHAVIOR

Preparing smaller portions and avoiding seconds are other "thin" eating habits recommended by The Federal Dietary Guidelines. You can be sure to prepare smaller portions by buying only enough food for smaller portions. You can avoid seconds by not having any available.

Behavioral psychologists have uncovered a number of other thin eating habits, not only at the table, but away from the table as well. Dr. Paul A. Thornton of the University of Kentucky is of the opinion that these practices are especially healthful in weight control and improving your enjoyment of daily life. To acquire some of these thin eating habits, follow these instructions.

• Avoid nibbling. One nibble has a negligible amount of calories. Many nibbles have enough calories to add a pound or more a week to your girth. Carry a pad and pencil with you, and jot down everything you nibble during one day. You may be so appalled at the amount of calories you consume, you'll stop nibbling cold-turkey. If not, jot down what you're planning on nibbling *before* you nibble. Chances are you'll lose your appetite.*

• Get over the idea that there are foods you're forbidden to eat. There's nothing more tempting than forbidden foods, and you're likely to binge on them. Follow the motto of The Federal Guidelines, everything in moderation, and enjoy a varied diet.

• Brush your teeth and rinse your mouth after eating. Much of the food you eat, particularly prepared foods, contain appetite stimulants (salt is one). Brushing your teeth and rinsing your mouth gets rid of these stimulants and ends after-meal hunger induced by them. (Of course, you know that brushing your teeth after meals fights tooth decay.)

• Serve restaurant-style, not family-style. The food on your plate is all you get, and you'll have no chance to help yourself to more.

• Eat your salad before your main dish. It's high in fiber, which expands in your stomach and leaves less room for the higher-caloric entrée.

---

*Nibbling refers here to food eaten in addition to regular meals. According to Dr. Thornton, if you replace meal calories with an equivalent amount of nibble calories, a metabolic change occurs that causes you to lose body weight at a faster rate.

• Eat only at one place in your home, preferably at your seat at the dining table. This eliminates eating in front of the TV, in your reading chair, in bed, in your workshop, and so on. One-place eating is a major calorie-cutter.

• Keep only a reasonable amount of ready-to-eat food in your home. What you don't have you can't eat.

• Keep ready-to-eat food in hard-to-get-to-places. If you have trouble getting to it, you won't take the trouble to get to it.

• Eat your snacks at the same time each day—and only then. That will cut down on between-meal snacking.

• Place this notice on your refrigerator door: DO NOT TAKE OUT FOOD EXCEPT AT REGULAR MEAL AND SNACK TIMES. That will reinforce your new eat-on-schedule-only habit.

• Eat without distractions. When you take your mind off what you eat, you overeat. Look what happens to you night after night in front of the tube.

• Shop for food after a meal, never on an empty stomach. When you're not motivated by hunger pangs, you'll shop sensibly. Otherwise, you'll overbuy, particularly high-caloric goodies.

• Shop for food with a shopping list—and stick to it. This will help blindfold you to the lure of supermarket displays.

• Avoid tasting more than once while cooking—and then only when the dish is almost ready. Every taste adds calories; and the more tastes, the fatter you'll get.

• Avoid chewing gum. It stimulates the salivary glands, and consequently the appetite.

• Avoid drinking carbonated beverages during a meal. The gas bloats your stomach, giving you a false sense of satisfaction. You eat less. Then, a short time after the meal, the bloat subsides, and you feel hungry.

All the behavior modifications leading to "thin" eating

habits that you've learned about so far apply whether you're on a reducing diet or a maintenance diet. But here are

SOME SPECIAL BEHAVIOR MODIFICATIONS TO HELP YOU LOSE WEIGHT

• Make a list of all the reasons you want to lose weight. Read the list before every meal and snack. Read the list when you're tempted to binge or stray.

• Become food-aware by keeping a diary and jotting down when and where and under what conditions you feel like breaking your diet. At the movies, watching TV, at a party? Or when you're unhappy, depressed, or when you feel like celebrating? At 11:00 A.M., 4:00 P.M., midnight? In this way, you'll find the mechanisms that trigger your over-eating. Once you're aware of them, you can find some means of making them ineffective. For example, if you find you eat when you're unhappy, try to cope with your emotional state some other way—making a telephone call to a friend, going for a walk, and so on. Your doctor can be of help to you in finding your overeating trigger mechanisms and suggesting ways to cope with them.

• On a sensible diet such as this one, don't weigh yourself daily. Fat loss ranges from one to two-and-a-half pounds a week, and after the first few days your scale may not indicate any change at all. A no-loss reading could discourage you. Weigh yourself once a week. Thus, weight loss is perceptible, and you'll be encouraged to continue. If your weight loss is only one pound a week, remember: that's fifty-two pounds a year. Be sure to weigh yourself naked without shoes at about the same time week after week. (Your body weight fluctuates as much as three pounds during the course of a day; so if you can't weigh yourself at the same time, you could get a false reading.)

• Scotch-tape to your full-length mirror a picture of yourself when you were thin. A shot in a bathing suit is preferable. Each day, compare with your undressed figure. That should provide strong motivation.

• Reward yourself each day for sticking to your diet—but not with food. Why not two tickets to that show you wanted to see, a new best seller, a long-distance call to the folks, and so on?

• Before you begin on your weight-reducing diet, take a picture of yourself, preferably in a bathing suit. Take another picture after four weeks. What a difference! Before and after photos are one of the strongest forms of motivation when you have to lose a great deal of weight.

• Never go to a party on an empty stomach.

• Get your mind off food by becoming more active mentally, physically and socially. Learning a new hobby has helped many people reduce.

• Plan for permanent weight loss, not just for looking attractive at a specific event. In this way, you'll learn lifetime weight-control habits that will help you keep your weight off once you've taken it off.

• Don't skip meals. That only sharpens your appetite. You're tempted to oversnack and/or overeat at your next meal. Particularly don't skip breakfast. Breakfast is so important to both a sound reducing and maintenance diet that we're devoting the following chapter to it.

8

How to Acquire the Breakfast Habit*

WHAT DO YOU EAT for breakfast? Nothing? A cup of coffee? Coffee with a doughnut or Danish?

You'll be amazed at how many people there are like you.

Bet the chances are small that you can reduce successfully or control your weight when you skip breakfast or have a coffee or a coffee-with breakfast. By midmorning or lunchtime, you'll be ravenous. Most breakfast-skippers are chronic overeaters.

The best way to acquire the breakfast habit is to understand why breakfast is so important to you, how you can enjoy a healthful breakfast even when you're in a hurry, how breakfast can become a highlight of your day with dishes you never thought of, how you can eat breakfast inexpensively and how you can enjoy hearty breakfasts without fear of gaining weight. We'll even tell you how to eat breakfast even though you're not hungry when you get up.

*The material in this chapter derives from "'Good Morning!' Breakfasts," which appears in the U.S. Department of Agriculture's publication *Food* (see footnote, page 46).

119

WHY BREAKFAST IS IMPORTANT TO YOU

Did you ever think about what the word "breakfast" means?

It means you've been fasting all night—and it's time to start refueling your body for the big day ahead. Food is the fuel your body needs to keep going. Refueling at breakfast helps many people to perform and feel better in the morning.

HOW YOU CAN ENJOY A HEALTHFUL BREAKFAST EVEN WHEN YOU'RE IN A HURRY

No time for breakfast? That's what many late risers say. But it isn't necessarily so! Check out these ways you can build a breakfast around foods that are ready-to-eat or take little preparation time.

Quick-to-fix foods

- Fresh, canned or frozen fruit and vegetable juices. Fresh and frozen juices can be prepared ahead and stored in the refrigerator.
- Fresh, canned or dried fruits.
- Milk, yogurt, cheese, cottage cheese, custard.
- Leftover poultry, fish and meat; canned fish, such as tuna.
- Leftover main-dish casseroles, such as macaroni and cheese.

- Breads, muffins, rolls, and the like.
- Quick-cooking and instant hot cereals.
- Ready-to-eat cold cereals.
- Frozen pancakes, waffles and French toast, homemade or bought.
- Quick breakfast drinks. Make drinks or shakes in a blender from milk and fruits or spices, such as cinnamon or nutmeg.

For those occasions when family members are late for work, foods that can be eaten along the way may mean the difference between breakfast—or no breakfast. Add one or two extras to your lunch bag that can be nibbled on the way to work or soon after you arrive.

Here are some foods you can eat on the go for breakfast:
- Fresh fruits, such as apples, bananas, oranges, strawberries or tangerines.
- Celery stuffed with peanut butter or a meat or cheese spread.
- Cherry tomatoes; strips of carrots, celery and green pepper; raw cauliflower or broccoli.
- Canned fruit or vegetable juices, fruits and puddings.
- Hard-cooked or deviled eggs. (Highly perishable foods, such as deviled eggs, chicken, meats and meat spreads, need to be kept refrigerator-cold if held for more than two to three hours before eating.)
- Cheese and crackers.
- Cold sliced meat loaf.
- Leftover chicken or turkey.
- Milk.
- Sandwiches. Some sandwich fillings can be prepared ahead of time. Try these combinations: Cottage cheese, shredded carrot, minced green pepper and tomato.
- Tuna, sliced green olives and salad dressing.

HOW BREAKFAST CAN BECOME A HIGHLIGHT OF THE DAY WITH DISHES YOU NEVER THOUGHT OF

You say you don't eat breakfast because breakfasts are so boring—the same thing day after day?

Why not try something new? Why not sautéed chicken livers for breakfast? Or a bowl of onion soup with grated cheese and crusty bread? There are many unconventional foods you could eat for breakfast that might be better for you than what you're eating right now. Try these—sometimes oddball—but really commonsense—ways to start out the day:

Cereals

There are plenty of ways to perk up cereals:

- Top cereals with favorite fruits—fresh in season or frozen, canned or dried. Try minted pineapple chunks, blueberries, cantaloupe or peach slices, figs; or a combination, such as bananas and strawberries.
- Add fruit, such as peach, apple, banana or pear slices or berries, to hot cereals.
- Stir chopped nuts, such as peanuts, pecans or walnuts, into cooked cereal.
- Make your own crunchy natural cereal (see page 181 for recipe). Serve it in a melon half.

Fruits and Vegetables

To make fruits and vegetables for breakfast more of an adventure:

- Serve a scoop of frozen yogurt or ice milk in a fruit juice.
- Top broiled or fried tomatoes with heated condensed mushroom soup.
- Top a cantaloupe half with cottage cheese or plain yogurt.
- Try a mug of hot tomato juice or tomato soup flavored with herbs, such as oregano or basil.
- Mix and chill fruits or fruits and a juice together, such as cantaloupe balls with strawberries and orange juice, berries with sliced peaches, sliced bananas with oranges.
- Broil a grapefruit half topped with fruit juice, such as cranberry or orange juice.
- Blend fruit juices such as pineapple juice and grapefruit juice, or cranberry juice and orange juice.
- Freeze fruit juices in an ice-cube tray to make juice cubes. Use juice cubes to chill other fruit juices.
- Drain canned peaches or pineapple, and heat under a broiler. Serve with breakfast meats.

Eggs

Try some of these ideas for a change of flavor:

- Combine any of the following with scrambled eggs— grated cheese, cottage cheese, fruit, such as orange sections or pineapple chunks, chopped onion, canned or cooked mushrooms, tomatoes, leftover potatoes, chopped ham or small sausages.
- For pizza eggs: Add a pinch of oregano, garlic powder or Italian seasoning, and either chopped black olives, mushrooms or cooked sausage, to eggs when scrambling. Spread tomato catsup on a toasted English muffin or toasted bread. Top with eggs and sprinkle with Parmesan cheese.

Other Foods

Here are some additional ideas you might want to try:

- For pancakes, try adding nuts, ham cubes, cooked sausage or fruits, such as bananas, strawberries, chopped apples, blueberries or crushed pineapple, to the batter.
- Add cinnamon or nutmeg to French toast batter.
- Make a breakfast sandwich using French toast or waffles with tomato slices, sliced bananas, sausage, ham, peanut butter or cheese between them.
- Sprinkle grated cheese over cooked waffles and broil.
- Split leftover rolls, biscuits, muffins or corn bread and toast in the oven. Put leftover roast beef, chicken or ham between halves of toasted rolls.
- Try a soup, such as clam chowder, split-pea or bean.
- Serve leftover cooked fish fillet, flaked and seasoned with Italian dressing, on whole-grain crackers.

HOW YOU CAN EAT BREAKFAST INEXPENSIVELY

Stretching food dollars in today's well-stocked markets can be a challenge, particularly for those on tight budgets. By careful selection, breakfast can be inexpensive and still furnish its share of the day's food. Some of the tips that follow may help you to economize on foods for breakfast as well as other meals.

- Check different forms of fruits and vegetables—fresh, canned, dehydrated, frozen—to see which is the best buy. Fresh foods in season will be at their peak in quality and are often low in cost.
- Watch for specials on canned and frozen products your

family likes. Stock up on good buys if you can store them properly.

- Try lower-priced brands of canned and packaged foods and those with no brand name shown (generic foods). You may like them as well as the more expensive ones. Store brands and generic foods may be similar enough in quality to widely known known products to satisfy you, yet cost less.
- Use unit pricing to find the brand or container size of food that costs the least per unit—pound, ounce or pint. (The unit price is usually shown on the shelf or above the compartment where the food is displayed in the store.) Even if it's a better buy, select a food only if you can store it properly and use it without waste.
- Limit purchases of perishable foods—even at bargain prices—to amounts that can be used while they are still good. The "pull date"—the last recommended day of retail sale—shown on some perishable foods may help you judge the freshness of the food when you buy it.
- Many ready-to-serve and instant hot cereals packaged as individual servings may cost two or three times as much per ounce as the same cereal in a larger box.
- Cereals you cook yourself are nearly always less expensive than the ready-prepared ones. Day-old bread and baked goods may be available at a great saving. Ask or watch for these in the stores where you shop.
- Many baked goods made at home cost less than ready-baked products.
- Buy fresh milk in half-gallon or one-gallon containers. Milk usually costs more purchased in small containers.
- Try nonfat dry milk in cooking and as a beverage. It costs only about one-half to two-thirds as much as an equal amount of fresh whole milk.
- Grated cheeses and wrapped cheese slices cost more than the same cheese in wedges or sticks.

- Cheeses in large boxes and jars, and cottage cheese in large cartons, cost less per pound or ounce than in smaller containers.
- Select from the cuts and types of meat, poultry and fish that provide the most cooked lean for the money spent.
- Check the "specials." At special prices, you may be able to afford some meat cuts that are usually beyond your budget.
- For low cost and variety in meals, use dry beans, dry peas, peanut butter and eggs some of the time in place of meat.

HOW YOU CAN ENJOY HEARTY BREAKFASTS WITHOUT FEAR OF GAINING WEIGHT

So many people skip breakfast because they feel it's a way to save calories—particularly when they think of breakfast in terms of pancake-and-sausage feasts. But sometimes being calorie-wise can be pound foolish. You've seen how often people who skip breakfast overeat at other meals because they're out-of-their-minds hungry.

Moderation is usually best in all things, particularly when you're on a diet. We offer these breakfast menus to help you get an idea of how foods add up in calories. The breakfasts range from 300 to 500 calories. A 500-calorie breakfast may seem like a lot of calories to have in the morning. But it isn't when you compare it with the 900 calories in a breakfast of 3 pancakes with syrup and margarine, 2 pork-sausage links and ½ cup of grapefruit juice.

THE I LOVE AMERICA DIET
BREAKFAST MENUS

Calorie values for individual foods are shown in parentheses.

300-Calorie Breakfasts

(1)

Vegetable-orange juice cocktail, ¾ cup (55)
(see recipe, page 170)
Plain cornflakes, 1 ounce, about 1⅛ cups (110)
with ½ cup skim milk (45)
Whole-wheat toast, 1 slice (65)
Jam, 1 teaspoon (20)
Coffee or tea without cream or sugar

(2)

Orange sections, ½ cup (45)
Potato-meat patty, 1 (175)
(see recipe, page 177)
Skim milk, 1 cup (90)
Coffee or tea without cream or sugar

(3)

Tomato juice, ¾ cup (35)
Scrambled egg, 1 (95)
Bran-cereal muffin (135)
Margarine, 1 teaspoon (35)
Coffee or tea without cream or sugar

400-Calorie Breakfasts

(1)

Grapefruit half (90)
Sandwich:
Tuna-vegetable filling, ¼ cup (125)
(see recipe, page 204)
Rye bread, 2 slices (120)
Skim milk, ¾ cup (65)

(2)

Cantaloupe, ¼ medium, 5 in. diameter (40)
Pork-sausage link, 1 ounce (60)
Poached egg, 1 (80)
Blueberry muffin, 1 (110)
Margarine, 1 teaspoon (35)
Low-fat milk (1 percent), ¾ cup (75)
Coffee or tea without cream or sugar

(3)

Pineapple juice, ½ cup (70)
Buttermilk toaster pancakes, 2, 4 in. diameter (180)
(see recipe, page 187)
with margarine, 1 teaspoon (35)
with syrup, 2 tablespoons (120)
Coffee or tea without cream or sugar

500-Calorie Breakfasts

(1)

Orange juice, ¾ cup (90)
Oatmeal, 1 cup (130)
with banana, one-half (50)
Whole-wheat toast, 1 slice (65)
with jam, 1 teaspoon (20)
Whole milk, 1 cup (150)

(2)

Canned pineapple chunks
in natural juice, ½ cup (70)
Sandwich:
Raisin toast, 2 slices (130)
Peanut butter, 2 tablespoons (190)
Low-fat milk (2 percent fat), 1 cup (120)

(3)

Honeydew melon, 1 wedge, 7 in. by 2 in. (50)
Red beans and rice, ½ cup (165)
(see recipe, page 190)
Pumpkin bread, 1 slice (200)
(see recipe, page 188)
Skim milk, 1 cup (85)

HOW TO EAT BREAKFAST EVEN THOUGH YOU'RE NOT HUNGRY WHEN YOU GET UP

There's no rule that says you *must* eat something *as soon as you get up*. You can always eat a little later in the morning. Late breakfasts are as good for you as early ones; and besides, they can be very fashionable!

If you don't eat breakfast because eating in the morning bothers you, start lightly with juice or a piece of fruit. Then, after several days, add bread or crackers. Then, later on, add a high-protein food such as milk, cheese, egg, peanut butter or meat. Before you know it, you will be a charter member of the "breakfast club."

Remember—for a good start in the morning and to help prevent you from overeating later in the day, our advice is eat *something*. Just juice is better than nothing at all. But a nutritious breakfast is best of all.

9

A Fitness Program from the President's Council on Physical Fitness and Sports

CONSISTENT EXERCISE is essential to your weight-reducing program and for staying fit for the rest of your life. This is how exercise helps keep you trim.*

CALORIES AND WEIGHT CONTROL

Calories are a measure of the energy food provides. How many calories you need to maintain your weight depends on how much energy you "burn" or use up.

Contrary to what many people believe, weight control shouldn't mean facing a lifetime of starvation and deprivation. Rather, the best way to manage your weight over a lifetime is to find a balance of proper nutrition, good food

*The material in this chapter is derived mainly from *Take the Time*, presented by the California Raisin Advisory Board and the President's Council on Physical Fitness and Sports, and on *Walking for Exercise and Pleasure*, developed by the President's Council on Physical Fitness and Sports, and published by Special Olympics, Inc

habits and regular exercise. Then, maintain your weight—if you go up a few pounds, increase your exercise and cut back on caloric consumption until you're back to the desirable weight.

To determine the number of calories needed to maintain your weight, follow this rule of thumb: For an adult, moderately active woman over twenty-two, multiply your desirable weight by fifteen calories/pound. (For example, a woman whose desirable weight is 120 pounds requires approximately 1,800 calories a day to maintain her weight.)

To lose weight, you must burn off about 3,500 extra calories, by dieting and/or exercise, to lose 1 pound of fat. Therefore, if you burn off 500 extra calories a day, you would lose 1 pound in a week. Slow, steady weight loss, one to two pounds per week, is healthier and more likely to be maintained.

The following "calorie costs" chart shows the approximate number of calories it takes to perform various activities, from sedentary to strenuous. A range of calories is given because body frame and weight affect the amount of calories used in any activity.

CALORIE COSTS

It takes:
- 80 to 100 calories per hour to perform SEDENTARY activities, such as reading, writing, watching TV, sewing or typing.
- 110 to 160 calories per hour for LIGHT activities, such as walking slowly, ironing or doing dishes.
- 170 to 240 calories per hour for MODERATE activities, such as walking moderately fast or playing table tennis.
- 250 to 350 calories per hour for VIGOROUS activities, such as walking fast, bowling, golfing or gardening.

• 350 or more calories per hour for STRENUOUS activities, such as swimming, tennis, running, dancing, skiing or football.

The more active you are, the more you can eat when you're reducing or maintaining your weight. Here are

MORE BENEFITS OF A FITNESS PROGRAM

- You'll discover joy and energy you never experienced before.
- You'll begin to develop a sense of yourself and your strengths.
- You'll delight in a sense of movement that you may have lost or may never have had.
- You'll look, feel and work better, and perhaps live longer.
- You'll increase your strength, endurance and co-ordination.
- You'll improve the functioning of your lungs, heart, blood vessels and digestive system.
- You'll minimize stress and release mental and physical tension.
- You'll reduce chronic fatigue. Physicians say that chronic fatigue is one of the classic symptoms of physical *unfitness*.

Physical fitness adds a new quality to your life—feeling fully alive. But simply "exercising" is not enough. In order to look and feel your best, a program involving a cardiovascular workout, flexibility, muscular endurance and muscular strength must be employed. Those are

THE FOUR MAJOR ELEMENTS OF A COMPLETE FITNESS PROGRAM

Cardiovascular Conditioning: With exercise, the heartbeat becomes stronger. Breathing becomes deeper and circulation improves. When circulation improves, you will find yourself with more energy and increased awareness. There also is evidence suggesting exercise decreases the risk associated with heart disease in both men and women. Dance/exercise, brisk walking, jogging and bicycle riding are examples of good exercises to strengthen the heart.

Flexibility: Muscles and other connective tissue lose elasticity with disuse. Joints need to be moved through their full range of motion. For many people, improved flexibility will reduce joint discomfort and lower-back pain and improve posture and personal appearance. Activities such as stretching exercises, dance and swimming will improve your flexibility.

Muscular Endurance: As your endurance increases, you will recover more quickly from vigorous activity and be able to exercise longer before tiring. You can build endurance through activities such as badminton, bicycle riding, canoeing, jogging, brisk walking and cross-country skiing.

Muscular Strength: Strength is essential for daily living, good posture and personal appearance. One of the best ways to achieve muscular strength is through weight lifting. However, calisthenics and dance/exercise also will help you build strength.

THE SIMPLEST AND BEST WAY TO START YOUR FITNESS PROGRAM—WALKING

Walking is easily the most popular form of exercise. Other activities generate more conversation and media coverage, but none of them approaches walking in number of participants. Approximately half of the 152 million American adults (18 years of age and older) claim they exercise regularly, and 2 of every 3 list walking as one of their activities. Nearly thirty-five million adults walk for exercise virtually every day and another fifteen million do so two or three times a week.

Walking is the only exercise in which the rate of participation does not decline in the middle and later years. In a recent national survey, the highest percentage of regular walkers (39.4 percent) for any group was found among men sixty-five years of age and older.

Unlike tennis, running, skiing, jogging and other activities that have gained great popularity fairly recently, walking has been widely practiced as a recreational and fitness activity throughout recorded history. Classical and early English literature seems to have been written largely by men who were prodigious walkers, and Emerson and Thoreau helped carry on the tradition in America. Among American Presidents, the most famous walkers included Jefferson, Lincoln and Truman.

Walking today is riding a wave of popularity that draws its strength from a rediscovery of walking's utility, pleasures and health-giving qualities.

THE ADVANTAGES OF WALKING

In some weight-loss and conditioning studies, walking actually has proved to be more effective than running and other more highly touted activities. That's because it's virtually injury-free and has the lowest dropout rate of any form of exercise.

Often dismissed in the past as being "too easy" to be taken seriously, walking has recently gained new respect as a means of improving physical fitness. Studies show that, when done briskly on a regular schedule, it can improve the body's ability to consume oxygen during exertion, lower the resting heart rate, reduce blood pressure and increase the efficiency of the heart and lungs. It also helps burn excess calories.

Since obesity and high blood pressure are among the leading risk factors for attack and stroke, walking offers protection against two of our major killers.

Walking takes longer to achieve the same results than do running and other more strenuous activities, but the difference is not as great as many people believe. A major university recently measured energy expenditure by four healthy male students during walks, jogs and runs of varying speeds. One of their findings: jogging a mile in 8½ minutes burns only 26 calories more than walking a mile in 12 minutes.

Walking conditioning effects improve dramatically at speeds faster than three miles per hour (twenty-minute miles). At that rate, the college student burned an average of 66 calories per mile. When they increased their pace to 5 miles per hour (12-minute miles), they used up 124 calories per mile. By way of comparison, they burned 164 calories per mile when running at 9 miles per hour.

Like other forms of exercise, walking appears to have a substantial psychological payoff. Beginning walkers almost invariably report that they feel better and sleep better, and that their mental outlook improves.

Walking also can exert a favorable influence on personal habits. For example, smokers who begin walking often cut down or quit. There are two reasons for this. One, it is difficult to exercise vigorously if you smoke; and two, better physical condition encourages a desire to improve other aspects of one's life.

Almost anyone can walk for exercise. You don't have to take lessons to learn how to walk. Probably all you need to do to become a serious walker is step up your pace and distance and walk more often.

You can walk almost anytime. You don't have to find a partner or get a team together to walk, so you can set your own schedule. Weather doesn't pose the same problems and uncertainties that it does in many sports. Walking is not a seasonal activity, and you can do it in extreme temperatures that would rule out other activities.

You can walk almost anywhere. All you have to do to find a place to walk is step outside your door. Almost any sidewalk, street, road, trail, park, field or shopping mall will do. The variety of settings available is one of the things that makes walking such a practical and pleasurable activity.

Walking involves almost no health risk. If you are free of serious health problems, you can start walking with confidence. But exercise good judgment and don't try to exceed the limits of your condition.

Walking doesn't cost anything. You don't have to pay fees or join a private club to become a walker. The only equipment required is a sturdy, comfortable pair of shoes.

WHAT MAKES A WALK A WORKOUT?

It's largely a matter of pace and distance. When you're walking for exercise, you don't saunter, stroll or shuffle. Instead, you move out at a steady clip that is brisk enough to make your heart beat faster and cause you to breathe more deeply.

Here are some tips to help you develop an efficient walking style:

- Hold head erect and keep back straight and abdomen flat. Toes should point straight ahead and arms should swing loosely at sides.
- Land on the heel of the foot and roll forward to drive off the ball of the foot. Walking only on the ball of the foot, or in a flat-footed style, may cause fatigue and soreness.
- Take long, easy strides, but don't strain for distance. When walking up or down hills, or at a very rapid pace, lean forward slightly.
- Breathe deeply (with mouth open, if that is more comfortable).

WHAT TO WEAR WHEN WALKING

A good pair of shoes is the only special equipment required by the walker. Any shoes that are comfortable, provide good support and don't cause blisters or calluses will do, but there are some suggestions to help you make your selection:

- Good running shoes (the training models with heavy soles) are good walking shoes, as are some of the lighter trail and hiking boots and casual shoes with heavy rubber or crepe rubber soles.
- Whatever kind of shoe you select, it should have arch supports and should elevate the heel one-half to three-quarters of an inch above the sole of the foot.
- Choose a shoe with uppers made of materials that "breathe," such as leather or nylon mesh.

Weather will dictate the rest of your attire. As a general rule, you will want to wear lighter clothing than temperatures seem to indicate. Walking generates lots of body heat.

In cold weather, it's better to wear several layers of light clothing than one or two heavy layers. The extra layers help trap heat, and they are easy to shed if you get too warm. A wool watch cap or ski cap will also help trap body heat and provide protection for the head in very cold temperatures.

WARMUP FOR WALKING

Walking is good exercise for the legs, heart and lungs, but it is not a complete exercise program. Persons who limit themselves to walking tend to become stiff and inflexible, with short, tight muscles in the back and backs of the legs. They may also lack muscle tone and strength in the trunk and upper body. These conditions can lead to poor posture and chronic lower-back pain, a problem that partially cripples or disables thousands of middle-aged and older Americans.

The exercises that follow are designed to increase flexibility and strength and to serve as a "warmup" for walking. Always do the exercises before walking.

STRETCHER Stand facing wall, arms' length away. Lean forward and place palms of hands flat against wall, slightly below shoulder height. Keep back straight, heels firmly on floor, and slowly bend elbows until forehead touches wall. Tuck hips toward wall and hold position for twenty seconds. *Repeat exercise with knees slightly flexed.*

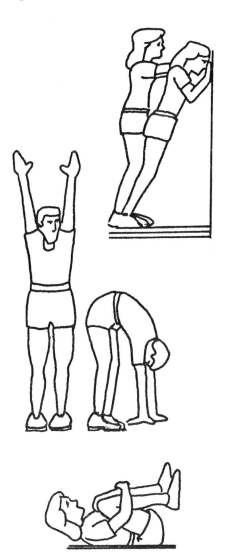

REACH AND BEND Stand erect with feet shoulder-width apart and arms extended over head. Reach as high as possible while keeping heels on floor and hold for ten counts. Flex knees slightly and bend slowly at waist, touching floor between feet with fingers. Hold for ten counts. (If you can't touch the floor, try to touch the tops of your shoes.) *Repeat entire sequence two to five times.*

KNEE PULL Lie flat on back with legs extended and arms at sides. Lock arms around legs just below knees and pull knees to chest, raising buttocks slightly off floor. Hold for ten to fifteen counts. (If you have knee problems, you may find it easier to lock arms behind knees.) *Repeat exercise three to five times.*

SITUP Several versions of the situp are listed in reverse order of difficulty (easiest one listed first, most difficult one last). Start with the situp that you can do three times without undue strain. When you are able to do ten repetitions of the exercise without great difficulty, move on to a more difficult version.

1. Lie flat on back with arms at sides, palms down, and knees slightly bent. Curl head forward until you can see past feet, hold for three counts, then lower to start position. *Repeat exercise three to ten times.*

2. Lie flat on back with arms at sides, palms down, and knees slightly bent. Roll forward until upper body is at 45-degree angle to floor, then return to starting position. *Repeat exercise three to ten times.*

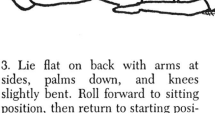

3. Lie flat on back with arms at sides, palms down, and knees slightly bent. Roll forward to sitting position, then return to starting position. *Repeat exercise three to ten times.*

4. Lie flat on back with arms crossed on chest and knees slightly bent. Roll forward to sitting position, then return to starting position. *Repeat exercise three to ten times.*

5. Lie flat on back with hands laced in back of head and knees slightly bent. Roll forward to sitting position, then return to starting position. *Repeat exercise three to fifteen times.*

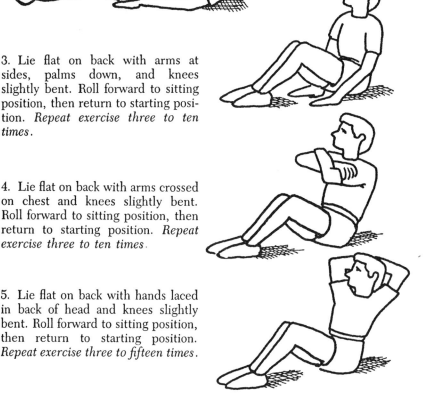

HOW FAR TO WALK, HOW FAST, AND HOW SOON YOU CAN DO IT

Now that you have decided to begin walking for exercise, you may be shocked at how poor your condition is. If at first you have difficulty in meeting the standards suggested here, don't be discouraged. You can systematically build your stamina and strength back to acceptable levels. Patience is the key to success. *Some experts say that it takes a month of reconditioning to make up for each year of physical inactivity.*

No one can tell you exactly how far or how fast to walk at the start, but you can determine the proper pace and distance by experimenting. We recommend that you begin by walking for twenty minutes at least four or five times a week at a pace that feels comfortable to you. If that proves to be too tiring, or too easy, reduce or lengthen your time accordingly.

Some very old people and some people who are ill begin by walking for one or two minutes, resting a minute and repeating this cycle until they begin to be fatigued. Where you have to start isn't important; it's where you're going that counts.

As your condition improves, you should gradually increase your time and pace. After you have been walking for twenty minutes several days a week for one month, start walking thirty minutes per outing. Eventually, your goal should be to get to the place where you can comfortably walk three miles in forty-five minutes, but there is no hurry about getting there.

The speed at which you walk is less important than the time you devote to it, although we recommend that you walk as briskly as your condition permits. It takes about twenty minutes for your body to begin realizing the "training effects" of sustained exercise.

The "talk test" can help you find the right pace. You should be able to carry on a conversation while walking. If you're too breathless to talk, you're going too fast.

The more often you walk, the faster you will improve. Three workouts a week are considered to be a "maintenance level" of exercise. More frequent workouts are required for swift improvement.

But listen to your body when you walk. If you develop dizziness, pain, nausea or any other unusual symptom, slow down or stop. If the problem persists, see your physician before walking again.

Don't try to compete with others when walking. Even individuals of similar age and build vary widely in their capacity for exercise. Your objective should be to steadily improve your own performance, not to walk farther or faster than someone else.

The most important thing is simply to set aside part of each day and *walk*. No matter what your age or condition, it's a practice that can make you healthier and happier.

HOW TO CHOOSE AN EXERCISE PROGRAM OTHER THAN WALKING

There's only one way to get in shape, and that's to get up, get going and start a fitness program for yourself—either through a class, or on your own.

Many people who exercise in groups find the professional leadership and social interaction the motivating factor to help them stay with their exercise program. Other people who may find they don't have time to go to a gym or class enjoy the quiet and privacy of their own home. Remember that not every exercise program is right for everybody, but one will feel comfortable to you.

You don't have to invent your own fitness program. There's lots of help at your local community center, "Y," or through adult education programs. There may be a program right where you work. More and more companies are adding "employee health and fitness programs" that offer professional staff, special facilities and exercise equipment. These programs are a tremendous help for someone just getting started. If you don't have an employee fitness program, talk with your employer about starting one.

GETTING STARTED

When beginning *any* exercise program, follow these tips:

1. It is advisable to have a medical checkup. If you have not had an examination in the past year, if you are past thirty, if you are overweight or if you have a history of high blood pressure or heart trouble, such an examination may help you to avoid extremely serious consequences.

2. Begin slowly, working up gradually. Even highly motivated individuals get discouraged when they exercise too vigorously too soon and develop unnecessary strain.

3. Start with five to ten minutes of bending and stretching to limber up muscles and get the heart and lungs going (see pages 139–140). In addition, allow five to ten minutes for a cool-down period at the end of the workout to allow your system to gradually return to a pre-stress condition.

4. Consistency is important to a fitness plan. Ideally, you should be exercising daily; however, try to work out at least four times a week—and vary your exercise. The amount of time you should exercise varies from person to person, but a

general recommendation is a minimum of twenty to thirty minutes.

AND—EXERCISE DURING YOUR WORKING HOURS

If you're on a physically active job, you don't have to. But if your only physical activity from nine to five is a stroll to the water cooler, you should.

The following exercises can be completed during your coffee break. They're good preparations for more vigorous activities after work or during weekends and vacations.*

1. *Half Head Turn:* Loosening up exercises, moves joints in the upper spinal column. Turn the head as far to the right as you can. Return head to the front. Turn head as far to the left as possible. Return head to the front. Repeat the whole exercise ten times.

2. *Head Tilt:* Loosening up exercise. Stimulates the neck muscles. Bend the head forward (with chin against throat) as far as possible. Bring the head slowly back as far as possible. Repeat the whole exercise ten times.

3. *Reach for the Sky:* Activates muscles in the shoulders. The shoulder muscles are stimulated by alternately and rhythmically stretching up the arms as if to pick a star from the sky. Repeat exercise ten times with each arm and shoulder.

4. *Stomach Bends:* Stimulates the bowels and blood circulation. In a sitting position, draw the stomach fully in. Drop the trunk forward while lifting the front of the feet high. Place the feet hard on the floor, relax the stomach muscles and raise upright slowly again. Repeat twenty times.

*These exercises were developed by the Governor's Council on Physical Fitness and Sports, Pennsylvania.

5. *Foot Patting:* Improves blood circulation to the feet and lower legs. Sit with elbows on knees, bend forward pressing your upper body down on your knees. Lift your toes with the heels as high as possible. Drop heels and lift toes. Repeat this exercise thirty times in its entirety.

6. *Partial Standing:* Improves knee and hip extension muscles. Slowly rise upward from sitting position without the help of the hands until you are standing erect. Sit down and repeat exercise twenty times.

7. *Cooling Down:* After completing these six exercises, sit fully relaxed. Breathe evenly and gently, counting slowly to thirty. Let the air out slowly and slowly take in deep breaths as you count. Repeat this exercise until you feel relaxed and comfortable.

These exercises will help improve muscle tone, flexibility and, to some extent, circulation. However, don't think you're ready for the four-minute mile if this is all you do. You *need* a *complete* fitness program.

10

Everything You Want to Know About Fats, Cholesterol, Sugar, Sodium, Fiber and the Basic Food Groups

THE NEW NUTRITION is based on your management of these nutrients and foods. It is only natural that you want to know more about them. This chapter amplifies the material supplied by The Federal Dietary Guidelines (Chapter 1).*

FATS

Fats in the diet come from two sources: (1) fats occurring naturally in foods such as whole milk, cheese, nuts, seeds, meat, poultry, fish, chocolate, and so on; and (2) fats and oils added in preparing foods such as fried foods, pastries, gravies, salad dressing, and so on.

All fats, no matter what the source (whether liquid oils,

*The information in this chapter is derived mainly from "People are Asking Questions About Sugar, Fat, Sodium and Fiber," which appears in *Food* (see footnote, page 46).

shortening, margarine, the marbling in meats or the fat in milk and cheese) have the same caloric value; however, saturated and polyunsaturated fats in diets differ in their effect on blood cholesterol; saturated fats elevate it.

To cut down on fat in your diet:
- Include more of these foods in your meals: fruits (except avocados and olives), vegetables, breads, cereals, dry beans and dry peas.
- Cut down on fatty meats. This includes regular ground beef, corned beef, spareribs, sausage and heavily marbled cuts, such as prime rib. Keep in mind that "prime" beef contains more fat than "choice," and "choice" more than "good" grade.
- Eat leaner cuts of meat, which include the following:
    Beef—flank, round, rump
    Lamb—leg, loin
    Veal—all cuts
    Pork—cuts such as lean ham, loin, Boston butt and picnic are moderate in fat content.
- Include more fish, shellfish, chicken and turkey in your diet. These foods are generally lower than many meats in fat content.
- Limit nuts, peanuts and peanut butter, which contain considerable amounts of fat.
- Reduce the use of whole milk and whole-milk products, such as most cheeses and ice cream, in favor of skim or low-fat milks and their products, such as uncreamed cottage cheese, which are lower in fat content.

CHOLESTEROL

People who eat a high-fat diet—especially a high-*saturated*-fat diet—often have higher levels of blood cholesterol. High levels of cholesterol (a fatlike substance) in the blood are linked to formation of fat deposits in the linings of arteries, a condition associated with heart disease. In contrast, diets with lower levels of fat and relatively more polyunsaturated fat (most vegetable oils) are linked to lower levels of blood cholesterol and possibly less risk of heart disease.

Cholesterol occurs naturally only in foods of animal origin. All meats contain cholesterol, which is present in both the lean and fat. The highest concentration is found in organ meats and in egg yolks. Fish and shellfish, except for shrimp, are relatively low in cholesterol. Dairy products also supply cholesterol.

SUGAR

Dietary sugar consists of a group of sweeteners. There's sucrose (cane and beet sugar), other caloric sweeteners, such as corn or glucose syrups, and sugars that occur naturally in foods—lactose in milk and fructose in fruit. The most common sweetener is table sugar (sucrose).

From 1960 to 1977, annual per capita consumption of caloric sweeteners increased about twenty-two pounds, mostly as a result of sweeteners added to commercially prepared foods and increased consumption of sweetened foods such as soft drinks. In addition to obviously sweet foods, such as candy, syrup, jam, jelly, pie and cake, many other commercially prepared foods and beverages contain substantial

CHOLESTEROL CONTENT
OF SELECTED FOODS
(in ascending order)

Food	Amount	Cholesterol
		Milligrams
Milk, skim, fluid, or reconstituted dry	1 cup	5
Cottage cheese, uncreamed	½ cup	7
Lard	1 tablespoon	12
Cream, light table	1 fluid ounce	20
Cottage cheese, creamed	½ cup	24
Cream, Half-and-Half	¼ cup	26
Ice cream, regular, approximately 10 per-cent fat	½ cup	27
Cheese, Cheddar	1 ounce	28
Milk, whole	1 cup	34
Butter	1 tablespoon	35
Oysters, salmon	3 ounces, cooked	40
Clams, halibut, tuna	3 ounces, cooked	55
Chicken, turkey, light meat	3 ounces, cooked	67
Beef, pork, lobster, chicken, turkey, dark meat	3 ounces, cooked	75
Lamb, veal, crab	3 ounces cooked	85
Shrimp	3 ounces cooked	130
Heart, beef	3 ounces, cooked	230
Egg	1 yolk or 1 egg	250
Liver, beef, calf, hog, lamb	3 ounces, cooked	370
Kidney	3 ounces, cooked	680
Brains	3 ounces, raw	more than 1700

SOURCE: *Fats in Food and Diet,* a publication of the Agricultural Research Service, U.S. Department of Agriculture.

amounts of sugars and sweeteners, even though they may not taste sweet. Catsup, salad dressings and peanut butter are examples.

Sugars and sweeteners play an important role in food preparation. Besides making foods taste good, they add texture and color to bakery products such as breads and pastries and help thicken, firm or preserve puddings, jellies, and the like.

Commonly eaten sugars and sweeteners offer little nutritionally except calories. When sugars and sweeteners make up a substantial share of your calories, they may replace other foods that offer vitamins, minerals and proteins in addition to calories. Because sweets are well liked, and contribute calories without bulk or fiber, it is easy to eat more of them—and more calories—than you realize.

More calories than you need make you fat. It doesn't matter where they come from, sugar or other sources.

Sweet foods, especially sticky sweets, are a major cause of dental cavities. Between-meal sweets (even cough drops) are worse offenders than the same foods eaten with meals. The total amount of sugar eaten is not as important as how many times, how long, and the form of sugary food (liquid or solid, for example) to which your teeth are exposed, and whether or not you clean your teeth after eating sugary foods.

Apart from sugar's role in tooth decay and its potential contribution to obesity, there is little evidence that directly links sugar with various disorders. However, scientists are still studying this issue.

To cut down on sugar in your diet:
• Check the ingredient label for sweeteners and sugars in products. Sugar is not the only word to look for on labels. Watch for such words as *sucrose, glucose, dextrose, fructose, corn syrups, corn sweeteners, natural sweeteners* and *invert sugar*. Remember that ingredients are listed on the label in

the order of predominance, with the ingredients used in largest amounts listed first.

• Substitute fruit juices or plain water for regular soft drinks, punches, fruit drinks and ades that contain considerable amounts of sugar.

• Go easy on candy, pies, cakes, pastries and cookies.

• Fruits are often canned in heavy syrup, which is a high-sugar product. Buy fruit canned in its own juice, other fruit juice or light syrup.

• Many cereals are presweetened. Check the label. Buy *unsweetened* kinds, so *you* can control the amount of sugar added.

• Experiment with reducing the sugar in your favorite recipes. Be prepared for dishes that may look and taste different, but can be equally as delicious, or more so, than those to which you are accustomed.

SODIUM

Excess sodium in the diet is believed to contribute to high blood pressure (hypertension) and stroke in some people. Excess sodium may also retain unnecessary amounts of water in the body. When sodium intake is decreased, this excess water may be excreted, resulting in rapid weight loss. In the opinion of the Department of Agriculture nutritionists, this water is later regained. But whether it will be regained on a consistently low-salt diet is disputed.

Excess water is associated with high blood pressure.

To cut down on your sodium intake, avoid:
• Foods prepared in brine, such as pickles, olives and sauerkraut.
• Salty or smoked meat, such as bologna, corned or chipped beef, frankfurters, ham, luncheon meats, salt pork, sausage, smoked tongue.

- Salty or smoked fish, such as anchovies, caviar, salted and dried cod, herring, sardines, smoked salmon.
- Snack items such as potato chips, pretzels, salted popcorn, and salted nuts and crackers.
- Bouillon cubes; seasoned salts (including sea salt); soy, Worcestershire and barbecue sauces.
- Cheeses, especially processed types.
- Canned and instant soups.
- Prepared horseradish, catsup and mustard.

Read labels. You may be surprised to learn that some processed foods that contain no table salt and don't taste salty have lots of sodium. Look for the words *soda* or *sodium* bicarbonate (baking *soda*), mono*sodium* glutamate (MSG), most baking powders, di*sodium* phosphate, *sodium* alginate, *sodium* sulfite and *sodium* saccharin.

SALT AND SODIUM CONVERSIONS

Grams to milligrams . . . . Multiply weight in grams by 1,000

Sodium into salt
(NaCl) equivalent . . . . Milligrams of sodium content
+ .40 = milligrams of salt

Salt into sodium . . . . Milligrams of salt × .40 = milligrams of sodium

Sodium in milligrams to sodium
in milliequivalents[1] . . . . Milligrams of sodium + 23 (atomic weight of sodium) = milliequivalents of sodium

Milliequivalents[1] of sodium to
milligrams of sodium . . . . Milliequivalents of sodium × 23 = milligrams of sodium

SOURCE: United States Department of Agriculture, *House and Garden Bulletin Number 233*, prepared by the Science and Education Administration in cooperation with Northeast Cooperative Extension Services.
[1]Medical prescriptions are often given as milliequivalents (mEq).

SALT AND CALORIE CONTENT OF SELECTED FOODS

Food	Salt content, mg	Calorie content
Cornflakes (1 cup)	251	97
Cocktail peanuts (1 cup)	132	838
Packaged white bread (1 slice)	117	62
Potato chips (10 chips)	191	113
Instant chocolate pudding (½ cup)	404	190
Dill pickles (1 large)	1,428	11
Tomato juice (1 cup)	486	46
Bacon (3 slices)	302	142
Beef broth (1 cup)	782	31
Milk (1 cup)	120	159
Bologna (1 lb)	5,897	1,379
Italian dressing (1 tbs)	314	83
Low-fat cottage cheese (½ cup)	459	152
Average hamburger & bun	1,510	360
Packaged American cheese (1 oz)	406	107
Catsup (1 tbs)	156	16
Peanut butter (1 tbs)	18	86
Chicken, white meat (1 lb)	377	394
Chicken, dark meat (1 lb)	377	313
Chili con carne with beans (1 cup)	1,354	339
Frankfurters (1 frankfurter)	499	140
Bun, frankfurter or hamburger (1 bun)	202	119
Apple pie (1 average wedge)	482	410
Ice cream (1 cup)	116	269
Beer (8-oz glass)	17	101
Watermelon (1 average slice)	6	156
Cheese pizza (1 average slice)	456	153

SOURCE: *Home and Garden Bulletin Number 233*, U.S. Department of Agriculture.

FIBER

Dietary fiber is plant material that is not digested in the human gastrointestinal tract. There are some indications that eating fibrous foods may prevent constipation and help prevent some chronic diseases of the large intenstine. In addition, fiber is a plus in weight reduction because bulky foods fill you up.

The types or amounts of fiber in foods that are the most beneficial to health are not known. However, plant foods—whole-grain breads and cereals, bran, dry peas and dry beans, nuts, fruits and vegetables, particularly those that are unpeeled or have edible seeds—are considered good sources.

THE BASIC FOOD GROUPS

1. Fruit-Vegetable Group

This group is important for its contribution of vitamins A and C and fiber, although individual foods in this group vary widely in how much of these they provide. Dark-green and deep-yellow vegetables are good sources of vitamin A. Most dark-green vegetables, if not overcooked, are also reliable sources of vitamin C, as are citrus fruits (oranges, grapefruit, tangerines, lemons), melons, berries and tomatoes. Dark-green vegetables are valued for riboflavin, folacin, iron and magnesium, as well. Certain greens—collards, kale, mustard, turnip and dandelion—provide calcium. Nearly all vegbles and fruits are low in fat, and none contains cholesterol.

Your diet should provide no fewer than four basic servings from this group daily. Include one good vitamin C source each day. Also frequently include deep-yellow or dark-green vegetables (for vitamin A), and unpeeled fruits and vegetables and those with edible seeds, such as berries (for fiber).

2. Bread-Cereal Group

These whole-grain or enriched foods are important sources of B-vitamins and iron. They also provide protein and are a major source of this nutrient in vegetarian diets. Whole-grain products contribute magnesium, folacin and fiber, in addition.

Most breakfast cereals are fortified at nutrient levels higher than those occurring in natural whole grain. In fact, some fortification adds vitamins not normally found in cereals (vitamins A, B-12, C and D). However, even these cereals, if refined, and other refined products (enriched or not), may be low in some other vitamins and trace minerals, which are partially removed from the whole grain in the milling process and are not added. For this reason, it's a good idea to include some less refined or whole-grain products in your diet.

Your diet should provide four basic servings from this group daily. Select only whole-grain and enriched or fortified products. But be sure to include *some* whole-grain bread or cereals. Check labels.

3. Milk-Cheese Group

Milk and most milk products are relied on to provide calcium (they're the major source of this mineral in the American diet) and riboflavin, and to contribute protein and vitamins A, B-6, and B-12. They also provide vitamin D, when fortified with this vitamin.

Fortified (with vitamins A and D), low-fat or skim-milk products have essentially the same nutrients as whole-milk products but fewer calories.

4. Meat-Poultry-Fish-Beans Group

These foods are valued for the protein, phosphorus, vitamins B-6, B-12, and other vitamins and minerals they provide. *However, only foods of animal origin contain vitamin B-12 naturally.*

It's a good idea to vary your choices among these foods, as each has distinct nutritional advantages. For example, red meats and oysters are good sources of zinc. Liver and egg yolks are valuable sources of vitamin A. Dry beans, dry peas, soybeans and nuts are worthwhile sources of magnesium. The flesh of fish and poultry is relatively low in calories and saturated fat. *Seeds (sunflower and sesame, for example) contribute polyunsaturated fatty acids,* which are an essential part of a balanced diet.

Remember—meats are reliable sources of iron. So are whole-grained and enriched breads and cereals, dry beans and dry peas; but the body can make better use of the iron these foods provide if they are eaten at the same time as a good source of vitamin C (orange juice, for example) or along with meat.

5. The Fifth Food Group

Fats, sweets and alcohol, with some exceptions, provide mainly calories. Vegetable oils generally supply Vitamin E and essentially fatty acids.

Fats and oils have more than twice the calories ounce for ounce as protein, starches or sugars, but help keep hunger pangs away longer.

Pure alcohol has almost twice the calories per ounce as protein, starches or sugars. However, few alcoholic beverages are 100 percent alcohol. Generally, the higher the alcohol content, the higher the calorie count, ounce for ounce.

Unenriched, refined bakery products are included in this group because they usually provide low levels of vitamins, minerals and protein compared with calories.

In general, the amount of fifth-group foods to use depends on the number of calories you require. As the basis of your daily diet, it's a good idea to concentrate first on the calorie-plus-nutrients foods provided in the other groups.

HOW TO READ A LABEL

Nutrition information on food labels can be used in making food selections. If a food label provides nutrition information, it must give:

- the size of a serving
- the number of servings in a container
- the number of calories and amount of protein, fat and carbohydrate (in grams) in a serving
- the amounts of eight nutrients—protein, vitamin A, thiamin, riboflavin, niacin, vitamin C, calcium and iron—in a serving expressed as a percentage of the U.S. Recommended Daily Allowance (U.S. RDA)

Information on nutrition labels can help you compare the nutritive value of different foods when following the Daily Food Guide and help you learn which foods are better sources of various nutrients (see page 163–165 for RDA's—Recommended Daily Allowances).

11

How The I Love America Diet Compares with the Average American Diet

BASIC NUTRITIVE VALUES

Nutrients	I Love America Diet	Average American Diet
FATS*	less than 35%	42%
SATURATED FATS	less than average	16%
CARBOHYDRATES*	50% or more (mostly complex)	46% (mostly simple)
PROTEIN*	15% or less	12%
CHOLESTEROL†	less than average	600–900
SUGARS†	less than average	18%
SODIUM†	1,100 to 3,000	2,300 to 6,900
FIBER	more than average	‡

SOURCE: *Facts About the Menus*, U.S. Department of Agriculture; *Dietary Goals for the United States*, Senate Select Committee on Nutrition and Human Needs; *The Sodium Content of Your Food*, U.S. Department of Agriculture; and *Fats in Food and Diet*, U.S. Department of Agriculture.

* In terms of total calories
† In milligrams
‡ No accurate figures available

HOW THE MAINTENANCE MENUS COMPARE WITH CURRENT CONSUMPTION PATTERNS

Fluid Milk and Yogurt

Recent surveys indicate that only half of the adults surveyed drink milk daily, with men using it more frequently than women.

The menus include fluid milk each day, and yogurt in one menu at both calorie levels.

The quantity of fluid milk and yogurt used in the menus is approximately the same as the per capita use of the population.

Cheese

Well over half the adults in recent surveys report using cheese one to six times a week. The menus include cheese four times.

Meat, Poultry and Fish

Over four fifths of adults report using meat and poultry once or twice a day, with women tending to have meat once a day.

With the exception of one lunch at the 1,600-calorie level, the menus offer meat, poultry or fish twice a day. The menus approximate the amount of beef and poultry as are consumed on a per capita basis. They appear to include slightly more fresh pork and somewhat less processed pork than presently consumed.

Eggs

Approximately two thirds of adults report using eggs one to six times a week.

The menus provide two to four eggs, both in recipes and as individual menu items.

Fruits and Vegetables

Most adults report having at least one serving of fruit or vegetable daily; fewer than one fifth report three or more servings of fruits and vegetables per day.

Fruits and vegetables in the menus are used both in recipes and as individual items, and substantially more servings of both are offered than are generally consumed.

Breads and Cereals (including pasta, rice, breakfast cereals, etc.)

Most adults report having one or two servings of bread, pasta, rice, etc., per day. Slightly over half rarely have breakfast cereals; the remainder generally have them one to six times a week.

The menus offer a variety of breads and cereals and use substantially more than is generally consumed. Breads and grain products are offered frequently at both calorie levels. Breakfast cereals are included on two menus.

Added Fats and Oils

On the average, the menus contain one half the amount of added fats and oils consumed on a per capita basis by Americans. The 1,600-calorie menus contain less fat than the 2,400-calorie menus. These fats and oils include salad dressings, margarine and cooking oil, but do not include the fats inherently found in foods such as milk, meats and nuts.

Added Sugars and Sweeteners (include cane and beet sugar, molasses, honey, corn syrup, etc.)

Average per capita sugar and sweetener consumption is estimated to be around 18 percent of calories.

The added sugar and sweetener content of the menus varies. The 1,600-calorie menus contain around a third, and the 2,400-calorie menus contain around half of the estimated sugar consumption on a per capita basis. The added sugar content of the menus depends in part on the choices made among beverage, dessert and snack options.

HOW THE NUTRIENT CONTENT OF THIS DIET COMPARES WITH RECOMMENDED DAILY ALLOWANCES (RDAs)

The menus in this diet generally meet or exceed recommended allowances for most nutrients. In diets of fewer than 1,800–2,000 calories, though, it is hard to get the recommended levels of all essential nutrients. That is particularly true of vitamins and minerals that are present in many foods but only in low concentrations. To approach the recommended levels of these nutrients at low-calorie levels, it is necessary to be more moderate in the use of fat, sugar and alcohol than many of us are accustomed to, and to eat more nutrient-dense foods.

Nutrient allowances are based on the Recommended Dietary Allowances developed by the Food and Nutrition Board, National Academy of Sciences, Washington, D.C. The allowances are revised periodically to reflect the latest scientific findings. The most recent RDAs, published in 1980, appear on the following chart.

RECOMMENDED DAILY DIETARY ALLOWANCES[a]

(Designed for the maintenance of good nutrition of practically all healthy people in the U.S.A.)

	Age (years)	Weight (kg)	(lb)	Height (cm)	(in)	Protein (g)	Fat-Soluble Vitamins		
							Vitamin A (µg RE)[b]	Vitamin D (µg)[c]	Vitamin E (mg α-TE)[d]
Infants	0.0-0.5	6	13	60	24	kg × 2.2	420	10	3
	0.5-1.0	9	20	71	28	kg × 2.0	400	10	4
Children	1-3	13	29	90	35	23	400	10	5
	4-6	20	44	112	44	30	500	10	6
	7-10	28	62	132	52	34	700	10	7
Males	11-14	45	99	157	62	45	1000	10	8
	15-18	66	145	176	69	56	1000	10	10
	19-22	70	154	177	70	56	1000	7.5	10
	23-50	70	154	178	70	56	1000	5	10
	51+	70	154	178	70	56	1000	5	10
Females	11-14	46	101	157	62	46	800	10	8
	15-18	55	120	163	64	46	800	10	8
	19-22	55	120	163	64	44	800	7.5	8
	23-50	55	120	163	64	44	800	5	8
	51+	55	120	163	64	44	800	5	8
Pregnant						+30	+200	+5	+2
Lactating						+20	+400	+5	+3

SOURCE: Food and Nutrition Board, National Academy of Sciences–National Research Council, Revised 1980

[a] The allowances are intended to provide for individual variations among most normal persons as they live in the United States under usual environmental stresses. Diets should be based on a variety of common foods in order to provide other nutrients for which human requirements have been less well defined.

[b] Retinol equivalents. 1 retinol equivalent = 1 µg retinol or 6 µg β carotene.

[c] As cholecalciferol. 10 µg cholecalciferol = 400 ɪᴜ of vitamin D.

[d] α-tocopherol equivalents. 1 mg d-α tocopherol = 1 α-TE.

RECOMMENDED DAILY DIETARY ALLOWANCES

(Designed for the maintenance of good nutrition of practically all healthy people in the U.S.A.)

Water-Soluble Vitamins

	Age (years)	Weight (kg)	Weight (lb)	Height (cm)	Height (in)	Vitamin C (mg)	Thiamin (mg)	Riboflavin (mg)	Niacin (mg NE)e	Vitamin B-6 (mg)	Folacinf (µg)	Vitamin B-12 (µg)
Infants	0.0-0.5	6	13	60	24	35	0.3	0.4	6	0.3	30	0.5g
	0.5-1.0	9	20	71	28	35	0.5	0.6	8	0.6	45	1.5
Children	1-3	13	29	90	35	45	0.7	0.8	9	0.9	100	2.0
	4-6	20	44	112	44	45	0.9	1.0	11	1.3	200	2.5
	7-10	28	62	132	52	45	1.2	1.4	16	1.6	300	3.0
Males	11-14	45	99	157	62	50	1.4	1.6	18	1.8	400	3.0
	15-18	66	145	176	69	60	1.4	1.7	18	2.0	400	3.0
	19-22	70	154	177	70	60	1.5	1.7	19	2.2	400	3.0
	23-50	70	154	178	70	60	1.4	1.6	18	2.2	400	3.0
	51+	70	154	178	70	60	1.2	1.4	16	2.2	400	3.0
Females	11-14	46	101	157	62	50	1.1	1.3	15	1.8	400	3.0
	15-18	55	120	163	64	60	1.1	1.3	14	2.0	400	3.0
	19-22	55	120	163	64	60	1.1	1.3	14	2.0	400	3.0
	23-50	55	120	163	64	60	1.0	1.2	13	2.0	400	3.0
	51+	55	120	163	64	60	1.0	1.2	13	2.0	400	3.0
Pregnant						+20	+0.4	+0.3	+2	+0.6	+400	+1.0
Lactating						+40	+0.5	+0.5	+5	+0.5	+100	+1.0

e I NE (niacin equivalent) is equal to 1 mg of niacin or 60 mg of dietary tryptophan.

f The folacin allowances refer to dietary sources as determined by Lactobacillus casei assay after treatment with enzymes (conjugases) to make polyglutamyl forms of the vitamin available to the test organism.

g The recommended dietary allowance for vitamin B-12 in infants is based on average concentration of the vitamin in human milk. The allowances after weaning are based on energy intake (as recommended by the American Academy of Pediatrics) and consideration of other factors, such as intestinal absorption.

RECOMMENDED DAILY DIETARY ALLOWANCES

(Designed for the maintenance of good nutrition of practically all healthy people in the U.S.A.)

	Age	Weight		Height		Minerals					
						Calcium	Phosphorus	Magnesium	Iron	Zinc	Iodine
	(years)	(kg)	(lb)	(cm)	(in)	(mg)	(mg)	(mg)	(mg)	(mg)	(µg)
Infants	0.0-0.5	6	13	60	24	360	240	50	10	3	40
	0.5-1.0	9	20	71	28	540	360	70	15	5	50
Children	1-3	13	29	90	35	800	800	150	15	10	70
	4-6	20	44	112	44	800	800	200	10	10	90
	7-10	28	62	132	52	800	800	250	10	10	120
Males	11-14	45	99	157	62	1200	1200	350	18	15	150
	15-18	66	145	176	69	1200	1200	400	18	15	150
	19-22	70	154	177	70	800	800	350	10	15	150
	23-50	70	154	178	70	800	800	350	10	15	150
	51+	70	154	178	70	800	800	350	10	15	150
Females	11-14	46	101	157	62	1200	1200	300	18	15	150
	15-18	55	120	163	64	1200	1200	300	18	15	150
	19-22	55	120	163	64	800	800	300	18	15	150
	23-50	55	120	163	64	800	800	300	18	15	150
	51+	55	120	163	64	800	800	300	10	15	150
Pregnant						+400	+400	+150	h	+5	+25
Lactating						+400	+400	+150	h	+10	+50

h The increased requirement during pregnancy cannot be met by the iron content of habitual American diets nor by the existing iron stores of many women; therefore the use of 30-60 mg of supplemental iron is recommended. Iron needs during lactation are not substantially different from those of nonpregnant women, but continued supplementation of the mother for 2-3 months after parturition is advisable in order to replenish stores depleted by pregnancy.

12

The I Love America Diet Recipes

ALL RECIPES WERE DEVELOPED in the laboratories of the Department of Agriculture and tested by a trained test panel to make sure they will meet with general approval.* Each recipe was designed for enjoyable eating while giving you a reasonable return in nutrients for the number of calories consumed.

Recipes have been catalogued under the four basic food groups to help you plan and keep track of the food-group quotas (Chapter 6). The four basic food groups are: Fruit-Vegetable, Bread-Cereal, Milk-Cheese and Meat-Poultry-Fish-Beans. In planning your daily menu, count a recipe as one selection toward a group quota. Some recipes will give you foods from more than one group, and some will give you foods from all groups; these are "bonus" recipes (but do not count them as more than one selection).

In developing the recipes in this chapter, the main goal of the U.S. Department of Agriculture nutritionists was to

*The recipes in this chapter appear in *Ideas For Better Eating*, published by the Science and Education Administration/Human Nutrition, U.S. Department of Agriculture, and in *Food*, published by the Consumer and Food Economics Institute, Human Nutrition Center, the Science and Education Administration, U.S. Department of Agriculture.

emphasize ingredients that provide nutrients. "At the same time, we tried to be practical," they reported. "If a food's too plain or too bland, you won't like it and you may not eat it. So we compromised. We tried to take it easy on added fat, sugar and salt—but we didn't *eliminate* them, because they add flavor and contribute to the texture of foods."

Let's take a brief look at how some of these delicious recipes have been made to conform to The Federal Dietary Guidelines.

• The apple crisp contains much less sugar than its traditional counterpart, and combines two whole-grain cereals for extra fiber.

• The bean salad calls for less oil than is often used.

• The Chinese-style vegetables call for less soy sauce than is customary. Soy sauce is virtually a saturated solution of salt.

• The chicken cacciatore cuts calories and fat by removing the skin; and herbs and spices are counted on for flavor, rather than salt and fat.

• The corn bread uses less salt and fewer eggs than usual, and calls for *stone-ground* cornmeal. The stone-grinding process preserves more of the nutrients in grain than any other milling process.

• The split-pea soup contains no added salt. There's already enough sodium in the ham or ham hock for flavor.

• The vegetable chowder offers a delectable way to increase the number and variety of vegetables in your diet. Whole-wheat flour is used as a thickener.

• The gingerbread is made with whole-wheat flour.

• The blueberry sauce is low in sugar, and has fewer calories than most pancake syrups.

• The eggnog has less fat and fewer calories than most.

• The brownies are made more nutritious by the addition of carrots and raisins. Pumpkin is added to the bread for the same reason.

These recipes avoid deep-fat-fried foods. As an alternative, you're introduced to stir-frying (page 220), a flavorful way to prepare low-calorie foods. More calories are cut by using mayonnaise-type salad dressing rather than mayonnaise itself. Several meatless main dishes are included, as well as whole-grain recipes. Fruits and vegetables are emphasized.

The dishes are the kind that most people like, and they rate four stars in their own right. But that doesn't mean they always taste the same as your own favorite version. Try them. Give yourself a chance to enjoy new tastes and flavors. The great bonus of the "new nutrition" is the new nutritious cooking—American style.

Use these recipes as a guide for adapting your own recipes to conform to The Federal Dietary Guidelines. For example, cut down on or eliminate the amount of salt, and see if your tastebuds approve; use low-fat or skim milk where a recipe calls for milk; replace high-fat dairy products with low-fat cheeses (low-fat cottage cheese or ricotta are just two); and reduce the amount of sugar used for sweetening. You'll be amazed at how light, refreshing and interesting your meals will become.

And if you don't have the time to cook, you'll find a bevy of quick and easy dishes for each food group, beginning on page 224.

The nutritionists at the Department of Agriculture recognize that people do not eat for nutritional benefits alone. Food must be appealing and enjoyable or no one will eat it, no matter how good it is for you. These recipes were developed to help make your mealtimes good times.

So eat and enjoy—new and familiar foods with perhaps a slightly different look or taste.

RECIPES FOR THE
FRUIT-VEGETABLE GROUP

ORANGE-PINEAPPLE CUP
4 servings, about ¾ cup each.
Calories per serving: about 145.

Orange sections	1 cup
Pineapple chunks, in own juice, undrained	8-ounce can
Seedless grapes	½ cup
Shredded coconut	½ cup
Mint leaves	if desired

1. Mix fruits and coconut together gently.
2. Chill until served.
3. Garnish with mint leaves.

PINEAPPLE COOLER
Makes 2 quarts.
Calories per 8-ounce cup: about 140.

Pineapple juice, unsweetened	46-ounce can
Lemon juice	2 tablespoons
Frozen orange juice concentrate	6-ounce can
Club soda, chilled	10-ounce bottle
Mint sprigs	if desired

1. Mix juices and frozen orange juice concentrate. Chill.
2. Add chilled club soda immediately before serving.
3. Serve over ice in tall glasses with straws. Garnish each serving with a sprig of mint, if desired.

ORANGE SMOOTHEE
6 servings, about ¾ cup each.
Calories per serving: about 115.

Frozen orange juice concentrate	6-ounce can
Milk	1 cup
Water	1 cup
Sugar	¼ cup
Vanilla	½ teaspoon
Ice cubes	10

1. Place all ingredients in a blender.
2. Cover and blend until smooth.
3. Serve immediately.

VEGETABLE-ORANGE JUICE COCKTAIL
10 servings, about ¾ cup each.
Calories per serving: about 55.

Vegetable juice cocktail	46-ounce can
Frozen orange juice concentrate	6-ounce can
Water	¾ cup
Basil leaves, crushed	1 teaspoon
Hot pepper sauce	3 drops

1. Mix all ingredients in a 2-quart container.
2. Chill thoroughly.

CRANBERRY TEA
6 servings, about 1 cup each.
Calories per serving: about 70.

Water	4 cups
Cloves, whole	12
Cinnamon sticks	2 short or 1 long
Sugar	2 tablespoons
Tea bags	4
Cranberry juice cocktail	2 cups

1. Place water, cloves, cinnamon sticks and sugar in a saucepan. Cover and bring to a boil.
2. Remove cinnamon sticks. Remove pan from heat.
3. Dip tea bags in the solution, cover and brew for 3 minutes, or longer if a stronger tea is desired. Remove tea bags.
4. Add cranberry juice cocktail. Return to a boil.
5. Serve hot in mugs.

FRUIT CUP
6 servings, about ⅔ cup each.
Calories per serving: about 95.

Frozen lemonade concentrate	3 tablespoons
Apple, cored, diced	1 medium
Orange, peeled, sectioned and diced	1 medium
Peach, pitted, diced	1 medium
Banana, peeled, sliced	1 medium
Seedless grapes, halved	½ cup
Blueberries	½ cup
Walnuts, finely chopped	2 tablespoons

1. Place lemonade concentrate in a large bowl and mix lightly with fruits as they are prepared. Chill.

2. Garnish each serving with chopped walnuts.

NOTE: Skins of apple and peach may be removed, if desired.

HOT FRUIT COMPOTE
6 servings, about ½ cup each.
Calories per serving: about 135.

Purple plums, drained	16-ounce can
Peach halves, drained	16-ounce can
Mandarin oranges	11-ounce can
Mandarin orange liquid	½ cup
Brown sugar, packed	2 tablespoons
Lemon rind, grated	½ teaspoon
Butter or margarine, melted	1 tablespoon

1. Preheat oven to 425°F (hot).
2. Place plums and peach halves in alternate layers in 1-quart baking dish.
3. Drain mandarin oranges; save liquid. Arrange oranges over fruits in baking dish.
4. Mix orange liquid, brown sugar.
5. Bake 30 minutes or until fruit is heated through.

BLUEBERRY SAUCE
4 servings, ¼ cup each.
Calories per serving: about 50.

Cornstarch	2 teaspoons
Water	½ cup
Frozen, unsweetened blue-berries, thawed, crushed	¾ cup
Honey	2 tablespoons
Lemon juice	2 teaspoons

1. Mix cornstarch with a small amount of water in a saucepan, stir until smooth.

2. Add remaining water, blueberries and honey.

3. Bring to boil over medium heat, stirring constantly. Cook until thickened.

4. Remove from heat. Stir in lemon juice.

5. Serve warm over whole-wheat pancakes (see recipe, page 182).

APPLE CRISP

4 servings, ½ cup each.
Calories per serving: about 250.

Tart apples, pared, sliced	4 cups
Water	¼ cup
Lemon juice	1 tablespoon
Brown sugar, packed	¼ cup
Whole-wheat flour	¼ cup
Old-fashioned rolled oats	½ cup
Ground cinnamon	½ teaspoon
Ground nutmeg	¼ teaspoon
Margarine	3 tablespoons

1. Place apples in 8 × 8 × 2-inch baking pan.

2. Mix water and lemon juice, pour over apples.

3. Mix sugar, flour, oats and spices.

4. Add margarine to dry mixture; mix until crumbly.

5. Sprinkle crumbly mixture evenly over apples.

6. Bake at 350°F (moderate oven) until apples are tender and topping is lightly browned, about 40 minutes.

MARINATED VEGETABLES
Makes 7 cups.
Calories per ½ cup: about 75.

Salad oil	⅓ cup
Cider vinegar	⅓ cup
Green pepper, finely chopped	2 tablespoons
Parsley, chopped	1 tablespoon
Salt	1 teaspoon
Paprika	¼ teaspoon
Pepper	⅛ teaspoon
Cauliflower, broken into florets, cooked tender-crisp	3 cups (1 small head)
Garbanzo beans, heated, drained	15-ounce can
Cucumber, unpared, sliced	2 cups
Carrots, cut in thin strips	1 cup

1. Place oil, vinegar, green pepper, parsley, salt and spices in a large bowl. Mix well.

2. Add vegetables. Mix gently.

3. Cover. Marinate for several hours or overnight in the refrigerator. Mix occasionally.

4. For optimum eating quality, use within a few days.

VEGETABLE CHOWDER

4 servings, about 1 cup each.

Calories per serving: about 150; with low-fat milk, about 125.

Onion, chopped	2 tablespoons
Celery, chopped	¼ cup
Green pepper, chopped	2 tablespoons
Margarine	1 tablespoon
Potatoes, pared, diced	½ cup
Water	1 cup
Marjoram, dried	¼ teaspoon
Salt	¼ teaspoon
Pepper	⅛ teaspoon
Corn, whole-kernel, frozen	1 cup
Green beans, cut, frozen	½ cup
Whole-wheat flour	2 tablespoons
Milk, whole or low-fat	1½ cups

1. Cook onion, celery and green pepper in margarine until almost tender.

2. Add potatoes, water and seasonings.

3. Cover and simmer until potatoes are tender, about 20 minutes.

4. Add corn and beans.

5. Cover and simmer 10 minutes longer, or until beans are tender.

6. Mix flour with a small amount of milk; add to remaining milk.

7. Stir milk mixture into cooked vegetable mixture.

8. Cook, stirring constantly, until slightly thickened.

VEGETABLE SOUP
6 servings, about ¾ cup each.
Calories per serving: about 80.

Oil	1 tablespoon
Green pepper, finely chopped	2 tablespoons
Onion, finely chopped	¼ cup
Celery, finely chopped	½ cup
Carrot, shredded	1 cup
Tomato soup, condensed	10¾-ounce can
Water	1¼ cups
Vegetable juice cocktail	12-ounce can

1. Heat oil. Add vegetables and cook until tender.
2. Mix tomato soup, water and vegetable juice cocktail in a saucepan. Bring to a boil.
3. Add vegetables. Cover and heat to serving temperature.
4. Serve in mugs.

FRUIT-NUT SNACK
Makes 3 cups.
Calories per tablespoon: about 35.

Spanish peanuts, salted	6½-ounce can
Raisins	1 cup
Dates, chopped	4 ounces

1. Mix ingredients.
2. Serve in small bowls.

POTATO-MEAT PATTIES
6 servings, 1 patty each.
Calories per serving: about 175.

Leftover mashed potatoes, seasoned	2 cups
Leftover meat, finely chopped	1 cup
Onion, finely chopped	2 tablespoons
Egg yolks	2
Milk	2 tablespoons
Pepper	⅛ teaspoon
Oil	2 tablespoons

1. Mix potatoes, meat, onion, egg yolks, milk and pepper.
2. Shape into 6 patties, using about ½ cup potato mixture for each.
3. Heat oil in frypan over moderate heat.
4. Cook patties until lightly browned on one side; turn and brown the other side.
5. Serve hot.

COTTAGE CHEESE STUFFED TOMATOES
6 servings, 1 tomato each.
Calories per serving: about 125.

Tomatoes, ripe	6 large
Cottage cheese, creamed or garden style	12-ounce carton
Salad dressing, mayonnaise-type	2 tablespoons
Pepper	⅛ teaspoon
Chives, chopped, dried	as desired
Lettuce cups	6

1. Wash and dry tomatoes. Remove cores.
2. Cut each tomato into wedges three-fourths of the way down. Pull apart slightly.
3. Mix cottage cheese, salad dressing and pepper.
4. Stuff tomatoes with the cottage cheese mixture.
5. Sprinkle with chives as desired.
6. Serve in lettuce cups.

VARIATION

TUNA STUFFED TOMATOES
Prepare tomatoes as above. Stuff with tuna salad (recipe on page 205 for French-toasted tuna sandwiches). About 175 calories per serving.

SQUASH BREAD
1 loaf, 16 slices.
Calories per slice: about 150.

Flour, unsifted	1½ cups
Cinnamon	2 teaspoons
Baking powder	1 teaspoon
Baking soda	½ teaspoon
Salt	¼ teaspoon
Eggs	2
Sugar	¾ cup
Oil	½ cup
Vanilla	2 teaspoons
Summer squash, coarsely shredded, lightly packed	1⅓ cups

1. Preheat oven to 350°F (moderate).
2. Grease a 9×5×3-inch loaf pan.
3. Mix dry ingredients *except sugar* thoroughly.

4. Beat eggs until frothy. Add sugar, oil and vanilla. Beat until lemon-colored, about 3 minutes.

5. Stir in squash.

6. Add dry ingredients. Mix just until dry ingredients are moistened.

7. Pour into loaf pan.

8. Bake 40 minutes or until toothpick inserted in center of loaf comes out clean.

9. Cool on rack. Remove from pan after 10 minutes.

CARROT-RAISIN BROWNIES

Makes 24 brownies, 2 by 2¼ inches each.
Calories per brownie: about 150.

Light brown sugar, packed	1½ cups
Butter or margarine, softened	½ cup
Eggs	2
Vanilla	1 teaspoon
Flour, unsifted	1½ cups
Salt	½ teaspoon
Baking soda	½ teaspoon
Baking powder	½ teaspoon
Raisins, chopped	½ cup
Carrots, finely grated	1½ cups
Walnuts, finely chopped	½ cup

1. Preheat oven to 350°F (moderate).

2. Grease a 9×13-inch baking pan.

3. Mix sugar and fat.

4. Add eggs and vanilla; beat.

5. Stir in dry ingredients. Add raisins and carrots; stir.

6. Spread mixture into baking pan; sprinkle with walnuts.

7. Bake about 40 minutes or until a toothpick inserted in center comes out clean.

8. Cool; cut into squares.

BANANA-NUT BREAD
1 loaf, 18 slices.
Calories per slice: about 135.

Whole-wheat flour	1¾ cup
Sugar	½ cup
Baking powder	1 tablespoon
Salt	¼ teaspoon
Walnuts, chopped	½ cup
Oil	⅓ cup
Eggs	2
Bananas, mashed	2 medium (about 1 cup)

1. Preheat oven to 350°F (moderate).
2. Grease 9 × 5 × 3-inch loaf pan.
3. Mix flour, sugar, baking powder, salt and nuts thoroughly.
4. Mix oil and eggs together. Mix in bananas.
5. Add dry ingredients to banana mixture. Stir until just smooth.
6. Pour into loaf pan.
7. Bake 45 minutes or until firmly set when lightly touched in center top.
8. Cool on rack. Remove from pan after 10 minutes.

RECIPES FOR THE
BREAD-CEREAL GROUP

CRUNCHY CEREAL
15 servings, about ½ cup each.
Calories per serving: about 280 with coconut; 290 with sunflower seeds.

Rolled oats, quick-cooking	3 cups
Unsweetened wheat germ	1 cup
Coconut, flaked or sunflower seeds, shelled	½ cup
Nuts, coarsely chopped	1 cup
Raisins	1 cup
Oil	½ cup
Honey	½ cup
Vanilla	2 teaspoons

1. Preheat oven to 275°F (very slow).
2. Mix rolled oats, wheat germ, coconut or sunflower seeds, nuts and raisins in a large bowl.
3. Mix oil, honey and vanilla. Pour over rolled-oat mixture. Stir lightly until evenly mixed.
4. Spread mixture on a 15 × 10 × 1-inch baking pan.
5. Bake 1 hour, stirring every 15 minutes.
6. Cool. Break up any large clumps. Store in an airtight container.

WHOLE-WHEAT PANCAKES *
4 servings, 2 pancakes each.
Calories per serving: about 245.

Whole-wheat flour	1⅓ cups
Baking powder	2 teaspoons
Salt	¼ teaspoon
Egg, slightly beaten	1
Milk	1⅓ cups
Brown sugar, packed	1 tablespoon
Oil	1 tablespoon

1. Grease griddle (see NOTE).

2. Heat griddle while mixing batter. Griddle is hot enough when drops of water sprinkled on it will bounce.

3. Mix flour, baking powder and salt.

4. Beat egg, milk, sugar and oil together.

5. Add liquid mixture to flour mixture. Stir only until flour is moistened. Batter will be slightly lumpy.

6. For each pancake, pour about ¼ cup batter onto hot griddle. Cook until covered with bubbles and edges are slightly dry.

7. Turn and brown other side.

NOTE: It is generally unnecessary to grease a well-seasoned griddle or one with a nonstick surface.

*For Blueberry Sauce, see page 172.

CEREAL PARTY SNACK
Makes 2 quarts.
Calories per ½ cup: about 225.

Butter or margarine	¼ cup
Worcestershire sauce	1 tablespoon
Hot pepper sauce	a few drops
Salted mixed nuts	12- to 14-ounce can
Pretzel sticks, short, thin	1 cup
Unsweetened, ready-to-eat	
cereals, assorted	4 cups
Paprika	1 teaspoon
Onion powder	¼ teaspoon
Garlic powder	dash

1. Preheat oven to 250°F (very slow).
2. Melt fat in a large baking pan in oven.
3. Remove pan from oven; stir Worcestershire and hot pepper sauces into melted fat.
4. Stir in nuts and pretzels; add cereals and mix well.
5. Sprinkle with seasonings; stir.
6. Heat uncovered in oven for 20 to 30 minutes, or until light-colored cereals begin to brown. Stir every 10 minutes.
7. Serve warm or cooled.
8. Store cooled cereal snack in tightly closed containers.
9. If snack needs recrisping, reheat in slow oven for a few minutes.

NOTE: Plain puffed cereals and bite-sized cereals can be used in this recipe.

HAM-CHEESE CRESCENT PINWHEELS
Makes 18 pinwheels.
Calories per pinwheel: about 35.

Refrigerated crescent rolls	4-ounce package (4 rolls)
Boiled ham, thinly sliced	2 slices, 4×6 inches, 1 ounce each
Prepared mustard	2 teaspoons
Pasteurized processed American cheese, shredded	⅓ cup (1½ ounce)
Caraway, sesame or poppy seeds	as desired

1. Preheat oven to 375°F (moderate).
2. Grease a baking sheet.
3. Unroll crescent dough and seal perforated seams.
4. Place ham slices on dough. Spread with mustard and sprinkle with shredded cheese.
5. Starting with the longer side, roll tightly and seal edges. Cut into 18 slices, about ¾ inch each.
6. Place pinwheels on baking sheet. Sprinkle with caraway seeds, sesame seeds, or poppy seeds, as desired.
7. Bake until lightly browned, about 12 minutes.

VARIATION

DATE-NUT CRESCENT PINWHEELS

Omit ham, mustard, cheese and seeds. Mix together ⅓ cup finely chopped pitted dates, 2 tablespoons finely chopped walnuts and 1 tablespoon orange juice. Spread mixture on unrolled crescent dough. Continue preparation as above. About 30 calories per pinwheel.

POPCORN WITH CHEESE
Makes about 6 cups.
Calories per cup: about 185.

Oil	¼ cup
Popcorn	⅓ cup
Butter or margarine, melted	2 tablespoons
Parmesan cheese, grated	½ cup
Salt, if desired	½ teaspoon

1. Preheat oven to 325°F (slow).
2. Place oil in a deep, heavy pan or skillet with a dome lid. Heat until oil is hot enough to pop a popcorn kernel.
3. Pour popcorn into pan. Cover and reduce heat to medium. Shake pan over the burner until all corn is popped.
4. Place popped corn in a shallow baking pan. Drizzle with melted fat. Mix.
5. Sprinkle with cheese. Add salt, if desired. Mix.
6. Heat 8 to 10 minutes in oven, stirring frequently.

NOTE: A popcorn popper may be used to prepare popcorn. Follow manufacturer's directions.

SNACK PIZZAS
Makes 10 pizzas.
Calories per pizza: about 105.

Refrigerator biscuits, flaky	9½-ounce package (10 biscuits)
Tomato paste	¼ cup
Oregano	1 teaspoon
Onion, chopped	¼ cup
Canned mushrooms, chopped	⅓ cup
Natural sharp Cheddar cheese, shredded	½ cup

1. Preheat oven to 400°F (hot).

2. Grease baking sheets.

3. Pat each biscuit round into a 4-inch circle on baking sheets.

4. Mix tomato paste and oregano. Brush on each biscuit round.

5. Mix onion and mushrooms. Sprinkle over tomato-paste mixture. Top with shredded cheese.

6. Bake until crust is lightly browned (about 8 minutes).

NOTE: Other ingredients, such as cooked ground sausage or ground beef, thin strips of salami, chopped green pepper or chopped anchovies may be used in place of onion and/or mushrooms.

SCONES
12 scones.
Calories per scone: about 145.

Flour, unsifted	2 cups
Sugar	¼ cup
Baking powder	2 teaspoons
Baking soda	½ teaspoon
Salt	½ teaspoon
Butter or margarine	¼ cup
Eggs	2
Sour milk (see NOTE)	⅓ cup

1. Preheat oven to 400°F (hot).

2. Grease a baking sheet.

3. Mix dry ingredients thoroughly.

4. Mix in fat *only* until mixture is crumbly. A pastry blender, two table knives or a fork may be used.

5. Beat eggs; add milk. Stir into dry ingredients. Mix just until moistened.

6. Divide dough in half. Place on baking sheet. Shape

each half of the dough into a 7-inch circle about ½-inch thick.

7. Cut each circle of dough into six wedges. Prick with a fork.

8. Bake 12 minutes or until lightly browned.

VARIATION

FRUIT SCONES

Add ½ cup chopped raisins or dates to egg-milk mixture. Proceed as in basic recipe. About 165 calories per serving with raisins or dates.

NOTE: To make sour milk, mix 1 teaspoon vinegar or lemon juice with enough sweet (regular) milk to make ⅓ cup. Let stand 5 minutes.

BUTTERMILK TOASTER PANCAKES

Twelve 4-inch pancakes.
Calories per pancake: about 90.

Eggs	3
Brown sugar, packed	1 tablespoon
Flour, unsifted	1 cup
Baking powder	1 tablespoon
Salt	½ teaspoon
Buttermilk	⅔ cup
Oil	2 tablespoons

1. Preheat griddle.

2. Beat eggs with brown sugar until very light, about 2 minutes.

3. Mix dry ingredients. Stir gently into beaten eggs.

4. Add buttermilk and oil. Stir only until mixed. Batter will be lumpy.

5. For each pancake, pour ¼ cup batter onto hot griddle.

6. Cook until surface is covered with bubbles, turn and cook other side until light brown.

7. Cool on rack.

8. Place pancakes in an airtight container with wax paper between layers. Or wrap singly in foil.

9. Label and store in freezer.

To reheat in toaster:

10. Remove from freezer and unwrap pancakes to be reheated.

11. Set toaster on medium-low setting.

12. Toast pancakes, twice if necessary, to heat through.

PUMPKIN BREAD

2 loaves, 16 slices each.
Calories per slice: about 200.

Flour, unsifted	4 cups
Sugar	3 cups
Baking soda	2 teaspoons
Salt	1½ teaspoons
Baking powder	1 teaspoon
Cinnamon	1 teaspoon
Nutmeg	1 teaspoon
Cloves	½ teaspoon
Ginger	¼ teaspoon
Pumpkin	16-ounce can
Oil	1 cup
Eggs	4
Water	⅔ cup

1. Preheat oven to 350°F (moderate).

2. Grease two 9×5×3-inch loaf pans.

3. Mix dry ingredients thoroughly in a large bowl.

4. Beat pumpkin, oil, eggs and water together. Add to dry ingredients. Stir just until dry ingredients are moistened. *Do not overmix.*

5. Pour one half of the batter into each loaf pan.

6. Bake 1 to 1¼ hours or until toothpick inserted in center of loaf comes out clean.

7. Cool on rack. Remove from pans after 10 minutes.

CORN BREAD

8 pieces, 2 × 4 inches each.
Calories per piece: about 220.

Stone-ground cornmeal (see NOTE)	2 cups
Baking powder	1 tablespoon
Salt	¼ teaspoon
Egg, slightly beaten	1
Milk	1 cup
Honey	2 tablespoons
Oil	¼ cup

1. Preheat oven to 400°F (hot).

2. Grease an 8 × 8 × 2-inch baking pan.

3. Mix cornmeal, baking powder and salt thoroughly.

4. Mix egg, milk, honey and oil. Add to cornmeal mixture.

5. Stir only until dry ingredients are moistened. Batter will be lumpy.

6. Pour into pan.

7. Bake 20 minutes or until lightly browned.

NOTE: Degerminated cornmeal may be used in place of stone-ground cornmeal.

RED BEANS AND RICE
6 servings, about ½ cup each.
Calories per serving: about 165.

Onion, chopped	½ cup
Celery, chopped	½ cup
Garlic	1 clove
Butter or margarine	2 tablespoons
Kidney beans	16-ounce can
Cooked rice	2 cups
Parsley, chopped	1 tablespoon
Salt	¼ teaspoon
Pepper	⅛ teaspoon

1. Cook onion, celery and garlic in fat until tender. Remove garlic.
2. Add remaining ingredients.
3. Simmer together for 5 minutes to blend flavors.

BAKED CHEESE GRITS
6 servings, about ⅔ cup each.
Calories per serving: about 230.

Salt	½ teaspoon
Water	2⅔ cups
Hominy grits, quick-cooking	⅔ cup
Butter or margarine	2 tablespoons
Pasteurized processed American cheese, shredded	1½ cups (6 ounces)
Eggs, beaten	2
Pepper	⅛ teaspoon

1. Preheat oven to 350°F (moderate).
2. Grease a 2-quart baking dish.

3. Add salt to water. Bring to a full, rolling boil. Add grits; return to boiling point. Cook, stirring constantly, until very thick, about 6 minutes.

4. Remove from heat. Add fat.

5. Mix cheese, eggs and pepper; stir into grits.

6. Pour into baking dish.

7. Bake 40 minutes or until lightly browned.

GINGERBREAD

8 servings, about 4×2 inches each.
Calories per serving: about 200.

Oil	½ cup
Water	½ cup
Molasses, light	⅓ cup
Sugar	⅓ cup
Egg whites, slightly beaten	2
Whole-wheat flour, unsifted	1 cup
Salt	¼ teaspoon
Baking powder	¼ teaspoon
Ginger	1 teaspoon
Cinnamon	½ teaspoon
Nutmeg	¼ teaspoon

1. Preheat oven to 350°F (moderate).

2. Grease lightly with oil and flour an 8×8×2-inch baking pan.

3. Mix oil and water. Add molasses, sugar, and egg whites. Stir until sugar is dissolved.

4. Mix flour, salt, baking powder, and spices. Add to liquid mixture. Beat until smooth.

5. Pour into pan.

6. Bake 30 minutes or until surface springs back when touched lightly.

RECIPES FOR THE MILK-CHEESE GROUP

COTTAGE CHEESE DIP
Makes 1¾ cups dip.
Calories per tablespoon: about 25.

Milk	2 tablespoons
Cottage cheese, creamed	12-ounce carton
Salad dressing, mayonnaise-type	¼ cup
Garlic powder	¼ teaspoon
Cayenne	dash
Onion salt	1 teaspoon

1. Place milk, cottage cheese, salad dressing, garlic powder, cayenne and onion salt in blender. Blend 1 minute or until cheese is smooth.
2. Pour mixture into a bowl. Cover and chill.
3. Serve with crisp vegetable sticks.

COTTAGE CHEESE-HERB DIP
Makes 1⅓ cups.
Calories per tablespoon: about 20.

Cottage cheese, creamed	1 cup
Lemon juice	2 tablespoons
Milk	2 tablespoons
Salad dressing, mayonnaise-type	2 tablespoons
Green onions, chopped	2 tablespoons
Parsley, coarsely chopped	¼ cup
Tarragon leaves	½ teaspoon
Pepper	Dash

1. Mix ingredients in a blender, scraping sides of blender jar with a rubber scraper and reblending as required until mixture is smooth and creamy.

2. Serve with fresh vegetable sticks.

CHILI CON QUESO DIP
Makes about 2½ cups.
Calories per tablespoon: about 35.

Pasteurized processed cheese spread, cut in cubes	16-ounce box
Canned tomatoes, chopped	¾ cup
Hot chili peppers, finely chopped	1 tablespoon

1. Place cheese cubes in the top of a double boiler over boiling water. Stir constantly until cheese is melted.

2. Stir in tomatoes and hot peppers until well blended and creamy.

3. Serve hot with tortilla or corn chips.

NOTE: Dip must be kept hot during serving in order to prevent excess thickening. A hot plate or chafing dish may be used.

BEEF AND CHEESE LOG
10-inch log, 40 ¼-inch slices.
Calories per slice without crackers: about 35.

Salad dressing, mayonnaise-type	1 tablespoon
Cream cheese, softened	3-ounce package
Natural sharp Cheddar cheese, finely shredded	1 cup (4 ounces)
Chopped pressed beef, finely chopped	3-ounce package
Pecans, finely chopped	½ cup

1. Mix salad dressing with softened cream cheese.
2. Add Cheddar cheese and beef. Mix well.
3. Shape into a 10-inch log. Roll in pecans.
4. Wrap in waxed paper. Chill.
5. Serve sliced with assorted crisp crackers.

EGGNOG

9 servings, about ½ cup each.
Calories per serving: about 160.

Eggs, slightly beaten	3
Sugar	½ cup
Salt	¼ teaspoon
Milk	3 cups
Half-and-half	1 cup
Vanilla	½ teaspoon
Imitation rum flavoring	1½ teaspoons
Nutmeg	as desired

1. Mix beaten eggs with sugar and salt in the top of a double boiler.
2. Add milk and half-and-half.
3. Cook over boiling water, stirring constantly, just until mixture coats spoon, about 10 to 15 minutes. Cool.
4. Add vanilla and rum flavoring. Chill.
5. Immediately before serving, strain eggnog. Beat with a rotary beater until frothy.
6. Pour into chilled cups. Sprinkle each serving with nutmeg, as desired.

NOTE: For this recipe, use only clean eggs, with no cracks in shells.

PEANUT BUTTER SUNDAE
6 servings, about ½ cup each.
Calories per serving: about 195.

Peanut butter, smooth	¼ cup
Honey	2 tablespoons
Milk	⅓ cup
Salt	a few grains
Vanilla ice milk	3 cups
Wheat germ	as desired

1. Stir peanut butter, honey, milk and salt together in a saucepan.

2. Cook over low heat, stirring constantly. Remove from heat when peanut butter is melted. Sauce should be smooth. Cool.

3. Serve sauce over ice milk. Sprinkle each serving with wheat germ, as desired.

STRAWBERRY-YOGURT POPSICLES
Makes 12 popsicles.
Calories per popsicle: about 70.

Frozen strawberries, thawed	2 cartons, 10 ounces each
Unflavored gelatin	1 tablespoon
Yogurt, plain	16 ounces
Paper cups, 3 ounce	12
Wooden sticks	12

1. Drain strawberries.

2. Place drained liquid in a saucepan and sprinkle with gelatin. Cook over low heat, stirring constantly, until gelatin dissolves.

3. Mix strawberries, yogurt and gelatin mixture in a blender until smooth.

4. Place cups on a tray or in a baking pan. Fill with blended mixture and cover cups with a sheet of aluminum foil.

5. Insert a stick for each popsicle by making a slit in the foil over the center of each cup.

6. Freeze popsicles until firm.

7. Run warm water on outside of cup to loosen each popsicle from the cup.

QUICK TOMATO RAREBIT
6 servings, ⅓ cup each.
Calories per serving: about 250.

Onion, finely chopped	¼ cup
Green pepper, finely chopped	2 tablespoons
Butter or margarine	½ tablespoon
Tomato soup, condensed	10¾-ounce can
Pasteurized processed sharp Cheddar cheese, shredded	2 cups (8 ounces)
Dry mustard	¼ teaspoon
Worcestershire sauce	¼ teaspoon
Toast, cut diagonally	6 slices

1. Cook onion and green pepper in fat until tender.

2. Heat soup in the top of a double boiler.

3. Add cheese to soup and cook over boiling water, stirring constantly, until cheese is melted and mixture is smooth.

4. Stir in mustard, Worcestershire sauce, onion and green pepper.

5. Serve over toast pieces. Garnish with a sprig of parsley, if desired.

BROILED PEAR AND SWISS CHEESE SANDWICH
6 servings, 1 sandwich each.
Calories per serving: about 205.

Sandwich bread	6 slices
Natural Swiss cheese slices	6 (1 ounce each)
Pears, pared, cored, sliced	2 medium
Sugar	1 tablespoon
Cinnamon	½ teaspoon

1. Toast bread.
2. Place a cheese slice on each piece of toast.
3. Arrange sliced pears on cheese.
4. Mix sugar and cinnamon. Sprinkle on pears.
5. Broil 10 minutes or until lightly browned.
6. Serve hot.

CHEESE FONDUE
6 servings, about ½ cup each.
Calories per serving: about 210 for fondue mixture, without bread.

Cottage cheese, creamed	1 cup
Milk	¼ cup
Butter or margarine	2 tablespoons
Cornstarch	1½ tablespoons
Garlic powder	dash
Dry mustard	¼ teaspoon
Milk	¾ cup
Pasteurized processed sharp Cheddar cheese, shredded	1 cup (4 ounces)
Pasteurized processed Swiss cheese, shredded	½ cup (2 ounces)
French bread, cut in cubes	1-pound loaf

1. Mix cottage cheese with ¼ cup milk in a blender until smooth.

2. Melt fat in a saucepan.

3. Stir in cornstarch, garlic powder and dry mustard; mix well.

4. Add ¾ cup milk. Cook over medium heat, stirring occasionally, until thickened, about 2 to 3 minutes.

5. Reduce heat. Stir in cottage cheese mixture.

6. Add remaining cheeses, stirring until cheeses are melted.

7. Serve with cubes of French bread for dipping into fondue mixture.

NOTE: Fondue may be transferred to a preheated fondue pot or chafing dish if desired. Keep hot during serving by using an alcohol burner, canned heat or candle burner.

QUICHE
8 servings.
Calories per serving: about 345.

Dried beef, coarsely cut	4 ounces
Butter or margarine	1 tablespoon
Pastry shell, unbaked, 9-inch	1
Natural Swiss cheese, coarsely shredded	1½ cups (7 ounces)
Pepper	¼ teaspoon
Dry mustard	⅛ teaspoon
Eggs	4
Half-and-half	1½ cups

1. Preheat oven to 375°F (moderate).

2. Lightly cook dried beef in fat, about 2 minutes. Cool slightly; sprinkle into pastry shell.

3. Sprinkle cheese over beef.

4. Mix seasonings and sprinkle over cheese.

5. Beat eggs and half-and-half together. Pour over cheese and beef.

6. Bake 40 minutes or until lightly browned and a knife inserted into the center comes out clean.

NOTE: If beef is very salty, pour 1 cup boiling water over beef. Drain well; then cut coarsely.

MACARONI AND CHEESE SOUFFLÉ

6 servings, 1 cup each.
Calories per serving: about 300.

Corkscrew-shaped macaroni	1½ cups
Butter or margarine	2 tablespoons
Flour	3 tablespoons
Salt	½ teaspoon
Paprika	½ teaspoon
Cayenne	dash
Milk	1¼ cups
Natural sharp Cheddar cheese, shredded	1½ cups (6 ounces)
Egg yolks	3
Egg whites	3

1. Preheat oven to 350°F (moderate).
2. Grease a 2-quart casserole.
3. Cook macaroni according to package directions.
4. Melt fat in a large saucepan.
5. Stir in flour, salt, paprika and cayenne.
6. Add milk. Cook over moderate heat, stirring until thickened.
7. Remove from heat. Add cheese and stir until melted.
8. Beat egg yolks until light. Add slowly to cheese sauce.
9. Add cooked macaroni.
10. Beat egg whites until stiff. Fold into macaroni and cheese mixture.
11. Pour into casserole.
12. Bake for 35 to 40 minutes or until center is firm to the touch when pressed lightly.
13. Serve immediately.

RECIPES FOR THE
MEAT-POULTRY-FISH-BEANS GROUP

RUMAKI
Makes 12 rumaki.
Calories per rumaki: about 30.

Chicken livers, washed, dried, halved	6
Horseradish mustard	1 tablespoon
Bacon slices, cut into thirds	4
Water chestnuts, cut in halves	6

1. Mix livers with horseradish mustard.
2. Wrap each bacon strip around a piece of liver and a water chestnut half. Secure with a toothpick.
3. Broil, turning frequently, until bacon is crisp, about 10 to 15 minutes.

NOTE: Use round wooden toothpicks for this recipe. Flat toothpicks may char during broiling.

ROSEMARY ALMONDS
Makes 2 cups.
Calories per tablespoon: about 55.

Almonds, whole, blanched	2 cups
Butter or margarine, melted	1 tablespoon
Salt	½ teaspoon
Cayenne	⅛ teaspoon
Rosemary leaves, crushed	2 teaspoons

1. Preheat oven to 350°F (moderate).
2. Mix all ingredients in a shallow pan.

3. Roast for 15 to 20 minutes, stirring occasionally, until lightly browned.

4. Drain on absorbent paper; cool.

TOASTED SUNFLOWER SEEDS

Makes 1 cup.

Calories per tablespoon: about 20 with oil; 15 without oil.

Sunflower seeds	1 cup
Oil, if desired	1 teaspoon
Salt, if desired	¼ teaspoon

1. Preheat oven to 325°F (slow).

2. Mix sunflower seeds with oil only if salt is used.

3. Spread plain or oiled seeds on baking sheet.

4. Bake about 8 minutes or until lightly browned. (Watch carefully, these seeds brown quickly.)

5. Sprinkle oiled seeds with salt while hot.

QUICK-COOK CHILI

6 servings, about ¾ cup each.

Calories per serving: about 270.

Ground beef	1 pound
Onion, chopped	½ cup
Pinto beans	16-ounce can
Tomato soup, condensed	10¾-ounce can
Chili powder	1 tablespoon, or as desired

1. Heat beef and onion in a frypan until beef is browned and onion is tender. Drain off excess fat.

2. Stir in remaining ingredients.

3. Cover. Simmer for 30 minutes, stirring occasionally.

SPLIT-PEA SOUP
6 servings, about 1 cup each.
Calories per serving: about 195.

Dry green split peas	1½ cups
Smoked ham hock	1 small
Onion, chopped	½ cup
Pepper	⅛ teaspoon
Water	6 cups

1. Add peas, ham hock, onion and pepper to water. Simmer, covered, 1½ hours or until ham hock is tender.

2. Remove ham hock and cut meat from bone. Cut meat into small pieces.

3. Return meat to soup. Heat to serving temperature.

OPEN-FACED EGG AND CHEESE SANDWICHES
Makes 6 sandwiches.
Calories per sandwich: about 300.

Butter or margarine	1 tablespoon
Onion, finely chopped	2 tablespoons
Green pepper, finely chopped	2 tablespoons
Eggs, beaten	6
Milk	⅓ cup
Salt	¼ teaspoon
Pepper	⅛ teaspoon
English muffin halves, toasted	6
Butter or margarine	about 1 tablespoon
Pasteurized processed American cheese	6 slices, 1 ounce each

1. Melt 1 tablespoon fat in a large frypan.

2. Add onion and green pepper. Cook until tender.

3. Mix eggs, milk, salt and pepper. Pour over onion and green pepper.

4. Cook over low heat, stirring occasionally to let uncooked portion flow beneath cooked portion. Continue cooking until eggs are set but still moist.

5. Divide into 6 portions.

6. Spread toasted muffin halves with 1 tablespoon butter or margarine.

7. Top muffin halves with egg mixture and a slice of cheese.

8. Broil until cheese is melted and lightly browned, about 5 minutes.

NOTE: For this recipe, use only clean eggs with no cracks in shells.

CHICKEN-VEGETABLE SANDWICH FILLING

1½ cups sandwich filling.

Calories per serving: about 100 for filling; 235 for a sandwich made with 2 slices of bread.

Chicken, cooked, finely chopped	1½ cups
Carrot, shredded	½ cup
Celery, shredded	½ cup
Onion, grated	4 teaspoons
Salad dressing, mayonnaise-type	¼ cup

1. Thoroughly mix all ingredients.

2. Chill.

3. Use about ¼ cup filling per sandwich.

VARIATION

TUNA-VEGETABLE SANDWICH FILLING

Use a 9¼-ounce can tuna in place of chicken. About 125 calories per serving for filling; 260 for a sandwich made with 2 slices of bread.

NOTE: Filling can be made the day before using. Store tightly covered in the refrigerator. Stir lightly before making sandwiches.

PEANUT BUTTER-ORANGE SANDWICH FILLING
2 cups sandwich filling.
Calories per serving: about 285 for filling; 420 for a sandwich made with 2 slices of bread.

Peanut butter, crunchy	1 cup
Honey	2 tablespoons
Salt	¼ teaspoon
Oranges, peeled, diced	1 cup

1. Thoroughly mix peanut butter, honey and salt.
2. Stir in oranges.
3. Chill.
4. Use about ⅓ cup filling per sandwich.

NOTE: Filling can be made the day before using. Store tightly covered in the refrigerator. Stir lightly before making sandwiches.

FRENCH-TOASTED TUNA SANDWICHES
Makes 6 sandwiches.
Calories per sandwich: about 360.

Tuna	9¼-ounce can
Celery, finely chopped	¼ cup
Onion, finely chopped	¼ cup
Sweet pickle relish	¼ cup
Salad dressing, mayonnaise-type	¼ cup
Bread, dry	12 slices
Eggs, beaten	2
Milk	⅓ cup
Vanilla	½ teaspoon
Oil or fat	about 2 tablespoons

1. Drain and flake tuna. Mix with celery, onion, relish and salad dressing.
2. Spread tuna mixture on 6 slices of bread; top with remaining slices.
3. Mix eggs, milk and vanilla.
4. Dip sandwiches into egg mixture to coat each side.
5. Brown in fat on a hot griddle or in a frypan, about 3 to 4 minutes on each side.

CHICKEN-FRUIT SALAD
6 servings, about 1 cup each.
Calories per serving: about 255.

Chicken, cooked, cut in chunky pieces	3 cups
Celery, chopped	¾ cup
Grapes, red, halved, seeded	¾ cup
Pineapple chunks in natural juice, drained	20-ounce can
Mandarin oranges, drained	11-ounce can
Pecans, chopped	¼ cup
Salad dressing	¼ cup
Salt	⅛ teaspoon
Lettuce leaves	as desired

1. Toss chicken, celery, grapes, pineapple, oranges and 3 tablespoons of the pecans together lightly.
2. Gently mix salad dressing and salt with chicken mixture. Chill.
3. Serve on lettuce leaves. Garnish with remaining pecans.

SALAD SUPREME
6 servings, about 1⅓ cups each.
Calories per serving: about 230.

Salad oil	2 tablespoons
Flour	1 tablespoon
Sugar	1 tablespoon
Prepared mustard	½ teaspoon
Water	¼ cup
Vinegar	¼ cup
Cooked ham, cut in thin strips	1½ cups

Onion rings	1 cup
Green pepper, cut in thin strips	½ cup
Cucumber, unpared, thinly sliced	1 cup
Celery, sliced	½ cup
Tomatoes, cut in thin wedges	2 cups
Lettuce, torn into bite-sized pieces	4 cups
Pasteurized processed American cheese, cut in thin strips	3 slices, 1 ounce each
Hard cooked eggs, sliced	2

1. For dressing, mix oil, flour, sugar, mustard, water and vinegar in a large frypan.

2. Cook over medium heat, stirring constantly until mixture comes to a boil.

3. Mix ham, onion, green pepper, cucumber and celery with dressing.

4. Cook covered over medium heat until heated through, about 4 to 5 minutes. Stir several times during cooking.

5. Remove from heat. Toss gently with tomatoes and lettuce.

6. Garnish with cheese strips and egg slices.

BEEF TACOS
6 servings, 2 tacos each.
Calories per serving without taco sauce: about 270. With sauce: about 340.

Taco shells, fully cooked	12
Ground beef	1 pound
Onion, chopped	¼ cup
Tomato sauce	8-ounce can
Chili powder	2 teaspoons
Tomato, chopped	1 cup
Lettuce, shredded	1 cup
Natural sharp Cheddar cheese, shredded	½ cup (2 ounces)
Taco sauce	as desired

1. Heat taco shells as directed on package.
2. Brown ground beef and onion in a frypan. Drain off excess fat.
3. Stir in tomato sauce and chili powder. Bring to a boil.
4. Reduce heat. Cook 10 to 15 minutes uncovered, stirring occasionally, until mixture is dry and crumbly.
5. Fill heated taco shells with approximately 2 tablespoons meat mixture.
6. Mix tomato, lettuce and cheese. Spoon about 2 tablespoons over beef in taco shells.
7. Drizzle with taco sauce, as desired.

VEGETABLE-NUT LOAF
6 servings, about 2½ × 4 inches each.
Calories per serving: about 450 with walnuts and 445 with pecans (not including sauce).

Wheat germ, unsweetened	to coat pan
Carrots, chopped	1 cup

Celery, chopped	1 cup
Onion, chopped	½ cup
Butter or margarine	¼ cup
Flour	¼ cup
Salt	1 teaspoon
Pepper	⅛ teaspoon
Thyme, if desired	¼ teaspoon
Milk	1½ cups
Natural Cheddar cheese, shredded	1 cup
Walnuts or pecans, chopped	1 cup
Wheat germ, unsweetened	¾ cup
Eggs, slightly beaten	3
Onion sauce	as desired

1. Preheat oven to 350°F (moderate).

2. Grease 8 × 8 × 2-inch baking pan. Coat with wheat germ.

3. Cook vegetables in fat until onion is tender.

4. Stir in flour, salt, pepper and thyme (if used). Stir in milk. Cook and stir over moderate heat until thick.

5. Stir in cheese, nuts and ¾ cup wheat germ. Add eggs.

6. Pour into baking pan.

7. Bake about 40 minutes or until well browned and firm.

8. Let stand a few minutes; cut into serving-size pieces. Serve with sauce.

ONION SAUCE FOR VEGETABLE-NUT LOAF
Makes 1½ cups.
Calories per ¼ cup: about 55.

Butter or margarine	2 tablespoons
Onion, finely chopped	2 tablespoons
Flour	¼ cup
Water or potato cooking liquid (see NOTE)	1½ cups
Soy sauce	2 teaspoons
Salt	½ teaspoon
Pepper	a few grains

1. Melt fat in small pan over moderate heat. Cook onion until lightly browned.
2. Stir in flour.
3. Remove from heat.
4. Stir in rest of ingredients. Cook and stir until thickened. Thin with a little water if needed.

NOTE: Broth from other cooked vegetables may be included.

ORIENTAL BEEF
6 servings, ¾ cup each.
Calories per serving: about 355 with rice.

Soy sauce	¼ cup
Cornstarch	2 teaspoons
Sugar	1 teaspoon
Ginger	½ teaspoon
Flank steak, trimmed, cut in 2 × ⅛-inch strips	1 pound
Vegetable oil	3 tablespoons
Green pepper, cut into thin strips	1 cup (about 1 medium)
Pineapple chunks, drained	20-ounce can
Cooked rice	3 cups (about 1 cup uncooked)

1. Mix soy sauce, cornstarch, sugar and ginger.
2. Coat meat with soy-sauce mixture.
3. Heat 1 tablespoon oil in a large frypan.
4. Add green pepper strips. Cook for 2 minutes, stirring constantly. Remove green pepper from pan.
5. Heat remaining 2 tablespoons oil.
6. Add meat. Cook for 1 to 2 minutes, stirring constantly, until beef is lightly browned.
7. Add green pepper and pineapple. Heat through.
8. Serve over rice.

NOTE: Steak is easier to cut when partially frozen.

FRANK KEBABS
6 servings, 1 kebab each.
Calories per serving: about 220.

Green pepper, cut into 12 squares	½ medium
Boiling water	About 1 cup
Onion, cut into 6 wedges	½ medium
Cherry tomatoes, stemmed	12
Potatoes, drained	1-pound can
All-meat franks, cut in thirds	6 franks, 2 ounces each
Barbecue sauce	½ cup

1. Cook green pepper squares in boiling water for 3 minutes.
2. Thread vegetables and franks onto six 12-inch skewers.
3. Brush with barbecue sauce.
4. Broil, occasionally basting with sauce, until browned. Turn and repeat for the other side, about 15 minutes total cooking time.

DEVILED CODFISH PATTIES
6 servings, 2 patties each.
Calories per serving: about 235.

Cod fillets, fresh or frozen	1½ pounds
Boiling water	1 cup
Salt	¼ teaspoon
Bread crumbs, soft	½ cup
Parsley, chopped	2 tablespoons
Salad dressing, mayonnaise-type	½ cup
Egg	1
Prepared mustard	1 tablespoon
Lemon juice	1 tablespoon
Worcestershire sauce	1 teaspoon
Pepper	⅛ teaspoon
Paprika	as desired

1. Thaw frozen fish.
2. Preheat oven to 400°F (hot).
3. Grease baking sheet.
4. Add fish to boiling, salted water. Cover and bring to a boil. Reduce heat and cook 4 minutes or until fish flakes easily. Drain and flake. Remove bones, if present.
5. Mix fish, bread crumbs and parsley.
6. Mix salad dressing, egg, mustard, lemon juice, Worcestershire sauce and pepper thoroughly. Stir into fish mixture. Mix well.
7. Form into 12 patties about 3 inches in diameter and ¾ inch thick on baking sheet.
8. Sprinkle with paprika.
9. Bake 15 to 20 minutes or until lightly browned.

LEMON BAKED FISH
6 servings, about 2 ounces each.
Calories per serving: about 130.

Flounder or haddock fillets, fresh or frozen	1 pound
Butter or margarine, melted	1 tablespoon
Lemon juice	4 teaspoons
Lemon rind, grated	1 teaspoon
Salt	⅛ teaspoon
Pepper	Dash
Rosemary	⅛ teaspoon

1. Thaw frozen fish.

2. Preheat oven to 350°F (moderate).

3. Divide fish into 6 servings. Place in single layer in a baking pan.

4. Mix fat, lemon juice, lemon rind, salt, pepper and rosemary. Pour over fish.

5. Bake for 25 minutes or until fish flakes easily when tested with a fork.

BROCCOLI-HAM ROLLUPS
6 servings, 1 rollup each.
Calories per serving: about 230.

Broccoli spears, frozen	2 packages, 10 ounces each
Butter or margarine	2 tablespoons
Flour	2 tablespoons
Salt	¼ teaspoon
Dry mustard	½ teaspoon
Milk	1 cup
Pasteurized processed sharp Cheddar cheese, finely shredded	1 cup (4 ounces)
Boiled ham, thinly sliced	6 inches, 1 ounce each

1. Preheat oven to 350°F (moderate).
2. Cook broccoli according to package directions until just tender.
3. While broccoli is cooking, melt fat in a heavy saucepan.
4. Stir in flour, salt and mustard.
5. Gradually stir in milk. Cook, stirring constantly, until thickened.
6. Add cheese and continue stirring until cheese is melted. Do not overcook.
7. Divide broccoli spears into 6 portions, splitting large stalks as necessary. Alternate direction of flower ends within each portion.
8. Place broccoli portions on and parallel to narrow end of each ham slice, extending flower ends over edges of ham.
9. Roll as for jellyroll with broccoli in the center of each rollup.
10. Arrange rollups in baking dish with seam side down.
11. Pour sauce over rollups. Bake until sauce is bubbly, about 20 minutes.

VARIATION
ASPARAGUS-HAM ROLLUPS

Use two packages of frozen asparagus spears in place of broccoli. About 225 calories per serving.

EGGS FU-YUNG
6 servings, 2 patties each.
Calories per serving: about 220.

Sauce

Chicken broth	1 cup
Soy sauce	2 tablespoons
Cornstarch	1 tablespoon
Water	¼ cup

Egg Mixture

Eggs	6
Pork, cooked, diced	1½ cups
Onions, small, thinly sliced	⅔ cup
Bean sprouts, drained	16-ounce can
Mushrooms, stems and pieces, drained	4-ounce can
Fat or oil	2 tablespoons

1. Mix broth and soy sauce. Heat to boiling.
2. Mix cornstarch and water. Stir slowly into the broth. Cook, stirring constantly, until thickened. Keep warm while cooking egg mixture.
3. Beat eggs until very thick and light.
4. Fold in pork, onions, bean sprouts and mushrooms.
5. Heat fat in frypan over moderate heat.
6. Pour egg mixture by ½ cupfuls into the pan.
7. Cook until lightly browned on one side; turn and brown the other side.
8. Serve sauce over the patties.

NOTE: For this recipe, use only clean eggs with no cracks in shells.

CREAMED CHICKEN
6 servings, about ¾ cup each.
Calories per serving: about 280 without patty shell, waffle or biscuit.

Butter or margarine	3 tablespoons
Flour	6 tablespoons
Milk	1½ cups
Chicken broth or stock	1½ cups
Salt	¾ teaspoon
Pepper	⅛ teaspoon
Ground savory	½ teaspoon
Cooked chicken, cut in pieces	2 cups
Peas, cooked	1 cup
Almonds, blanched, slivered	½ cup

1. Melt fat in a large saucepan; stir in flour.
2. Mix in liquids and seasonings.
3. Cook over moderate heat, stirring constantly, until smooth and thickened.
4. Add chicken, peas and almonds. Continue cooking until heated through.
5. Serve hot in patty shells or over toasted waffles or biscuits.

VARIATION

CREAMED TUNA

Use two 7-ounce cans of solid water-packed tuna, drained, in place of chicken, and use ½ cup coarsely chopped cashews in place of almonds. Omit salt and savory. About 270 calories per serving.

OPEN-FACED SUBMARINE SANDWICHES
Makes 6 sandwiches.
Calories per sandwich: about 285.

English muffin halves, toasted	6
Butter or margarine	about 1 tablespoon
Salami slices, cut into quarters	6 slices, 1 ounce each
Lettuce, chopped	1 cup
Onion, thinly sliced and separated into rings	½ small
Tomato, thinly sliced	1 medium
Basil leaves	½ teaspoon
Pasteurized processed American cheese	6 slices, 1 ounce each

1. Spread toasted muffin halves with butter or margarine.
2. Layer salami quarters, lettuce, onion and tomato slices on toasted muffin halves.
3. Sprinkle with basil.
4. Top each sandwich with cheese slice.
5. Broil until cheese is melted and is lightly browned, about 5 minutes.

PICKLED EGGS
Makes 6 eggs.
Calories per egg: about 80.

Juice drained from canned beets	about ¾ cup
Vinegar	¾ cup
Brown sugar	¼ cup
Salt	½ teaspoon
Cloves, whole	12
Eggs, hard cooked, peeled	6

1. Mix beet juice, vinegar, brown sugar, salt and cloves in a saucepan. Bring to a boil. Cool.

2. Place eggs in a quart jar. Add beet juice mixture.

3. To keep eggs immersed in the pickling mixture, fill a small plastic bag (intended for food use) with water; fasten securely to prevent leakage; and place on top of eggs.

4. Refrigerate overnight.

5. For optimum eating quality, use within 2 days after preparation.

BEAN SALAD
4 servings, ¾ cup each.
Calories per serving: about 280.

Kidney beans, canned, drained	1 cup
Garbanzo beans, canned, drained	1 cup
Carrots, very thinly sliced	½ cup
Onion, chopped	¼ cup
Sweet pickle, chopped	3 tablespoons
Salt	¼ teaspoon
Pepper	⅓ teaspoon
Dry mustard	½ teaspoon
Vinegar	3 tablespoons
Honey	1 tablespoon
Oil	¼ cup

1. Mix vegetables and pickle in a bowl.
2. Thoroughly mix remaining ingredients.
3. Pour over vegetable mixture. Mix gently.
4. Chill at least 1 hour before serving.

FLOUNDER FLORENTINE

4 servings, about 3 ounces fish and ¼ cup spinach each.
Calories per serving: about 140.

Frozen skinless flounder fillets, thawed	1 pound
Boiling water	1½ cups
Frozen chopped spinach	10-ounce package
Onion, finely chopped	1 tablespoon
Marjoram	½ teaspoon
Flour	2 tablespoons
Skim milk	1 cup
Salt	½ teaspoon
Pepper	dash
Grated Parmesan cheese	2 tablespoons

1. Place fish fillets in 1 cup boiling water. Cook, uncovered, 2 minutes. Drain.

2. Place spinach and onion in ½ cup boiling water. Separate spinach with fork.

3. When water returns to boiling, cover and cook spinach 2 minutes. Drain well. Mix with marjoram.

4. Put spinach in 8×8×2-inch glass baking dish. Arrange cooked fish on top of spinach.

5. Mix flour thoroughly with ¼ cup of milk.

6. Pour remaining milk in saucepan. Heat.

7. Add flour mixture slowly to hot milk, stirring constantly. Cook, stirring constantly, until thickened. Stir in salt and pepper.

8. Pour sauce over fish. Sprinkle with Parmesan cheese.

9. Bake at 400°F (hot oven) until top is lightly browned and mixture is bubbly, about 25 minutes.

BEEF WITH CHINESE-STYLE VEGETABLES
4 servings, ½ cup of meat and ½ cup vegetables each.
Calories per serving: about 200.

Beef round steak, lean, boneless	1 pound
Green beans, cut in strips	⅔ cup
Carrots, thinly sliced	⅔ cup
Turnips, thinly sliced	⅔ cup
Cauliflower florets, thinly sliced	⅔ cup
Chinese cabbage, cut in strips	⅔ cups
Boiling water	⅔ cup
Oil	2 teaspoons
Cornstarch	4 teaspoons
Ground ginger	½ teaspoon
Garlic powder	⅓ teaspoon
Soy sauce	1 tablespoon
Sherry*	3 tablespoons
Water	½ cup

1. Trim fat from beef. Slice beef across the grain into thin strips, about ⅛ inch wide and 3 inches long. (It is easier to slice meat thinly if it is partially frozen.)

2. Add vegetables to boiling water. Simmer, covered, for 5 minutes or until vegetables are tender but still crisp. Drain.

3. While vegetables are cooking, heat oil in nonstick frypan. Add beef and stir-fry over moderately high heat, turning pieces constantly until beef is no longer red, about 2 to 3 minutes.

---

*Sherry may be omitted if desired. Use 3 tablespoons water in place of sherry. About 185 calories per serving when made without sherry.

4. Mix cornstarch, garlic powder, ginger, soy sauce, sherry and water.

5. Stir cornstarch mixture into beef. Heat until sauce starts to boil.

6. Serve meat sauce over vegetables.

CHICKEN CACCIATORE
4 servings, one-half breast each.
Calories per serving: about 155.

Onion, chopped	½ cup
Boiling water	¼ cup
Tomatoes	8-ounce can
Tomato purée	½ cup
Garlic clove	1
Oregano leaves	1 teaspoon
Celery seed	½ teaspoon
Pepper	⅓ teaspoon
Chicken breast halves, without skin	4

1. Cook onion in boiling water until tender. Do not drain.

2. Add tomatoes, tomato purée, garlic, oregano, celery seed and pepper to onions. Simmer 10 minutes to blend flavors.

3. Place breast halves in heavy frypan. Pour tomato mixture over chicken.

4. Cook, covered, over low heat until chicken is tender, about 60 minutes.

5. Remove garlic clove before serving.

CHILI BEAN DIP
Makes 1⅓ cups.
Calories per tablespoon: about 15 without vegetable sticks.

Kidney beans, drained	16-ounce can
Vinegar	1 tablespoon
Chili powder	¾ teaspoon
Ground cumin	⅓ teaspoon
Onion, very finely chopped	2 teaspoons
Parsley, chopped	2 teaspoons
Raw vegetable sticks	as desired

1. Place drained beans, vinegar, chili powder and cumin in blender. Blend until smooth.
2. Remove mixture from blender. Stir in onion and parsley.
3. Serve with raw vegetable sticks.

SPICY BAKED FISH
4 servings, about 2½ ounces fish each.
Calories per serving: about 110.

Cod fillets, fresh or frozen, without skin	1 pound
Onion, chopped	¼ cup
Green pepper, chopped	¼ cup
Oil	2 teaspoons
Tomatoes	8-ounce can
Salt	¼ teaspoon
Pepper	⅓ teaspoon

1. Thaw frozen fish.
2. Grease 9×9×2-inch baking pan lightly with ½ teaspoon of oil.

3. Cut fish in 4 servings. Place in baking pan.

4. Bake at 350°F (moderate oven) until fish flakes easily, about 20 minutes. Drain cooking liquid from fish.

5. While fish is baking, cook onion and green pepper in remaining oil until onion is clear.

6. Cut up large pieces of tomatoes.

7. Add tomatoes, salt and pepper to cooked onion and green pepper.

8. Cook 20 minutes to blend flavors.

9. Pour sauce over drained fish.

10. Bake 10 minutes.

13

The I Love America Diet Fast Foods and Snacks

IN THIS CHAPTER, you'll find fast foods listed for the four basic food groups. Keeping "servings" in mind, use them to round out your reducing or maintenance menus on those occasions when you don't have the time or you're just not in the mood to cook something more elaborate. There's a section here on snacks as well—and some of them will pleasantly surprise you.*

FAST FOODS

THE FRUIT-VEGETABLE GROUP

- Apples, peaches, pears, grapes, etc.
- Raw vegetable sticks or pieces (radishes, celery, cauliflower, green onions, zucchini, green pepper, carrots, cucumbers—even parsnips!).
- Dried apricots, raisins, prunes.
- Canned fruits or fruit juices, kept chilled in the refrigerator.

*This chapter is derived mainly from "Is It True What They Say about Snacking?" and "Quick and Easy," both of which appear in *Food*, see footnote, page 46.

- Ripe tomatoes—eat 'em right out of your hand!
- Mini-kebabs of bite-sized fruit chunks, strung on a toothpick.
- Banana chunks dipped in orange juice. Shake in a bag with chopped peanuts. Spear with toothpicks.
- Celery stuffed with cottage cheese, cheese spread or peanut butter.
- Juice cubes you make by freezing fruit juice in an ice-cube tray. Chill other fruit drinks with them.
- Chilled cranberry juice mixed with club soda. Grape-fruit half, sprinkled with brown sugar and broiled.
- Tomato half, sprinkled with bread crumbs, Parmesan or grated Cheddar cheese, and broiled. Creative salads of lettuce, raw spinach and other fresh vegetables, fruits, meats, eggs, or seafood.

THE BREAD-CEREAL GROUP

- Raisin bread, toasted and spread with peanut butter.
- Sandwiches using a variety of breads—raisin, cracked-wheat, pumpernickel, rye, black.
- Date-nut roll or brown bread, spread with cream cheese.
- English muffins, served open-faced for sandwiches such as hot roast beef or turkey, chicken salad, sloppy joes.
- Individual pizzas. Top English muffin halves with cheese slices, tomato sauce and oregano, and broil.
- Waffles topped with whipped topping and strawberries.
- Wheat or rye crackers, topped with herb-seasoned cottage cheese, cheese or meat spread, or peanut butter.
- Graham crackers and milk.
- Ready-to-eat cereals—right out of the box.
- Ice cream or pudding, sprinkled with crisp cereals or wheat germ.

THE MILK-CHEESE GROUP

- Milkshakes with mashed fresh berries or bananas.
- Parfait of cottage cheese, yogurt or ice milk, combined with fruit, sprinkled with chopped nuts, wheat germ or crisp cereal.
- Dips for vegetable sticks. For fewer calories, substitute cottage cheese or plain yogurt for sour cream and mayonnaise in preparing dips.
- Fruit-flavored yogurt.
- Cheese cubes, *au naturel,* or speared with pretzel sticks, or alternated with mandarin orange sections on a toothpick.
- Assorted cheeses with crackers or chilled fresh fruits.
- Custard or pudding.
- Ice-milk sundae, topped with fresh, canned or frozen fruits.

THE MEAT-POULTRY-FISH-BEANS GROUP

- Nuts, sesame seeds or toasted sunflower seeds.
- Sandwich spread of peanut butter combined with raisins or chopped dates.
- Peanut butter and honey spread on an English muffin, sprinkled with chopped walnuts and heated under broiler.
- Grilled open-faced peanut butter and mashed banana sandwich.
- Tomatoes stuffed with egg salad.
- Melon wedges topped with thinly sliced ham.
- Sandwiches of cheese, meat, tomato, onion and lettuce.
- Antipasto of tuna, shrimp, anchovies, hard-cooked eggs and assorted vegetables.
- Leftover poultry or meat—as is, or chopped into a sandwich spread.
- Bite-sized cubes of broiled beef, served on a toothpick.

SNACKS

Ever since you were a kid, you've probably heard that snacks are bad for you.

Are they?

Well, yes. *And* no. Yes, if you gobble up foods that are loaded with sugar, salt and fat, but low on protein, vitamins and minerals. But, if you use snacks to supply your body with nutritious foods that your regular meals are lacking, then snacking is a great idea. Keeping your eye on your main goal—a *balanced* diet—is most important of all.

What should you eat for snacks on a maintenance diet? You can't go wrong stocking up with foods like fresh fruits, juices, yogurt, milk, cheese, nuts, whole-grain or enriched crackers and other foods from the four basic food groups. These foods make great snacks and contribute to the day's need for nutrients. The fast foods in this chapter are also favorites of many snackers.

Sometimes you may need a snack to take the place of a regular meal with all the trimmings. Then you need a bigger snack than usual—not just a few nuts or an apple, but something more substantial—like a sandwich, a bowl of chili or pizza. Now you're in the ballpark of what we call a "small meal." Small meals usually provide more food value than most snacks but do not require a lot of accompanying foods and often do not take as long to fix as a regular full-course meal. Small meals can sometimes be hearty and provide lots of calories—like a Dagwood sandwich, or they can be light on calories—like a salad. Like snacks, the type of small meal that is right for you depends on *who* you are, and *what* you do.

Keep ingredients on hand for spur-of-the-moment small meals. Ground beef, eggs, cheese, vegetables, breads and pasta are basic ingredients with which you can do a lot.

Foods you can prepare ahead of time and have on hand in the freezer will also help out when the occasion calls for a small meal. Buy ground beef, shape into individual patties and freeze. Freeze homemade casseroles, chili, soups and pizza. Make up double recipes of pancakes or waffles, then freeze the extras. Make and freeze your own TV dinners from extra servings of food made at regular meals. Even partially prepared ingredients can help out in a pinch. Chop and freeze onions and green peppers; make bread crumbs and cracker crumbs; grate, wrap and refrigerate cheese for casserole toppings.

Casseroles, chili, pizza and pancakes? Sure, we're still talking about "snacks." It's just that we've come a long way since cookies and milk!

HOW TO SNACK ON A REDUCING DIET

If you're overweight, remember that food by any name is still food, and lots of little snacks can add up to big trouble (even if nobody sees you eat them!). You could avoid snacks altogether—but here's a better idea: *Plan snacks as part of your total allotted calories for the day*. Use the reducing menus as guidelines. Snacks average 25 to 50 calories a day.

But how can you tell when other snacks are low-calorie?

Here are some guidelines:

As a general rule, food is likely to be relatively low in calories if it is:*

- thin and watery—like tomato juice
- crisp but not greasy-crisp—like celery, radishes, cu-

*Adapted by the U.S. Department of Agriculture from "Food Needs and Energy Use in Weight Reduction," by Ruth M. Leverton, *Journal of the American Dietetic Association*, vol. 49, pp. 23–25, 1966.

cumbers, melons and many other fresh fruits and vegetables
- bulky—like salad greens

A food is likely to be relatively high in calories if it is:
- greasy-crisp or oily—like fried tidbits and other fried foods, butter, margarine
- smooth and thick—like rich sauces, cream cheese, peanut butter, cream
- sweet and gooey—like candy, regular soft drinks, rich baked goods, and other desserts
- alcoholic

Be snack-wise and you won't feel deprived when you see other people nibbling.

Come to think of it, be I Love America Diet-wise, and you won't feel deprived food-wise any time in your life.

14

Up-to-date Tips for Dieters

As THIS BOOK was going to press, the American Dietetic Association published *Food 2—Getting Down to Basics: A Dieter's Guide*. Instrumental in the development of the *Guide* was the United States Department of Agriculture's Human Nutrition Service. The *Guide* doesn't tell you how to diet, but it does review up-to-date facts about weight loss and supplies commonsense tips for weight control. Here are some highlights from *Food 2*.

If your family and friends tell you to "eat today and diet tomorrow," enlist their support by making them understand your anxieties and goals. Then they'll be on your side, encouraging and helping you to diet successfully.

If you're confused about initial fast weight loss and subsequent slower weight loss on the same amount of calories, here's a clarification. During the first weeks of calorie reduction, a *temporary* readjustment of water balance in the body results in water-weight loss in addition to fat loss. Once your body adjusts to the new lower calorie intake, your weight loss due to water excretion may slow down. Fat loss is slower than water loss.

If you stop losing weight after the first few weeks on a

230

diet even though you continue to cut calories, you may be eating too much salty food such as ham, cheese, and pickles. This causes mild fluid retention, which adds weight. Another reason for your failure to lose weight is that since you're thinner you need fewer calories. Cut down *further* on your calories, and you'll continue to lose weight.

If you're a refrigerator raider, stick to raw vegetables as snacks.

If you bake and taste, bake on a full stomach so you won't be tempted.

If the sight of small portions is unsatisfying, serve on smaller plates to make the portions look larger.

If you want to eat more slowly to cut your intake of food, one way is to eat the kind of food you have to work at, like oranges. It takes more time to eat an orange than to drink a glass of orange juice.

If you eat in fast-food places, select milk instead of a milkshake, a small plain burger or lean beef sandwich instead of a "jumbo" with all the trimmings. Go easy on batter-coated deep-fried chicken and fish; they're relatively high in calories.

If you think there are negligible calories in condiments, look at the facts. One tablespoon of catsup plus one tablespoon of sweet pickle relish contain forty calories. Condiment calories can add up.

If you've been searching for a "different" kind of low-calorie meal, why not try a vegetable sandwich made up of whole-wheat pocket bread with sliced cucumbers, tomatoes, green pepper rings, bean sprouts, mushrooms and watercress, moistened with plain low-fat yogurt seasoned with curry or garlic?

If you're afraid that exercise will increase your appetite and prevent weight loss, the President's Council on Physical Fitness and Sports reminds you that moderate exercise does *not* increase the appetite of obese people.

If you don't like formal exercise, why not use the stairs instead of the elevator, park at the far end of the parking lot and walk the rest of the way, stand instead of sitting when you use the phone, do household chores like vacuuming or mowing the lawn, and avoid the drive-up bank—walk inside instead?

If your child is chubby, ask your doctor or dietitian to work out and supervise a weight-control program that takes into consideration the child's special nutritional needs while growing. Because of those needs, children's weight-control programs often maintain—not reduce—weight. Good eating habits and plenty of support from you and your family will help your child grow into a trim adult. The best way to have your children avoid weight problems is to set a good example of weight control yourself.

If you think you can go back to your old ways of eating and exercising after you've reached ideal weight, you're wrong; that's the way to gain back the pounds you've lost. It takes determination to stay at your ideal weight, but it can be done when you continue your new eating and exercise habits.

Food 2 also contains an analysis of several types of fad diets, sample low-calorie menus (1,200, 1,500, and 1,800 calories per day), and a cooking section of numerous low-calorie recipes. *Food 2* is available from The American Dietetic Association, 430 North Michigan Avenue, Chicago, Illinois 60611 (312) 280-5022. Write or call for price information.

Also available from the same source is *Food 3—Eating the Moderate Fat and Cholesterol Way,* a guide to moderating the total fat, saturated fat, and cholesterol in your diet— a goal considered sensible by many scientists, including the Surgeon General of the United States.

A Personal Note
from Phyllis George

You've read this book, and now you're standing on the threshold of a new life for yourself.

It can be an excitingly successful life.

That's because a healthy attitude spells success, and a healthy attitude depends on a healthy body.

If you feel wonderful, you'll perform wonderfully day after day, no matter how tough the jobs ahead of you.

But a healthy body means discipline. Don't be careless. Don't make excuses. Don't let the future slip away from you.

A healthy body and a healthy attitude have brought me many accomplishments. But I know the best part of my life is still ahead of me. I'm looking forward to many new successes.

So can you.

I want to live a long, healthy life, be a good partner to my husband, and a good mother always. I know I can do it.

So can you.

I want to be high all the time with the joy of living, with working and playing, with being with people. I'm doing it, and I'll continue to do it.

So can you.

But it's up to *you*. Nobody can do it except you. Nobody's responsible except you. Nobody but *you* can make it happen.

Start today to make it happen.

With the *I Love America Diet*.

—PHYLLIS GEORGE BROWN

Lexington, Kentucky
Summer, 1982

Recommended Reading

The Changing American Diet (1978) by Letitia Brewster and Michael F. Jacobson, Ph.D. (Center for Science in the Public Interest, 1755 S Street, N.W., Washington, D.C. 20009).

Nutrition (1981) by Cheryl Corbin (Holt, Rinehart & Winston, 383 Madison Avenue, New York, N.Y. 10017).

A Diet for Living (1975) by Jean Mayer, Ph.D. (David McKay, 750 Third Avenue, New York, N.Y. 10017).

The Prudent Diet (1981) (Bureau of Nutrition, New York City Department of Health, 93 Worth Street, Room 714, New York, N.Y. 10013. Free when request is accompanied by a stamped, self-addressed envelope).

Obesity in America (1979) edited by Dr. George A. Bray (Public Health Service, National Institutes of Health, Department of Health and Human Services [formerly Department of Health, Education and Welfare], Federal Building, 7550 Wisconsin Avenue, Bethesda, Maryland 20205).

Vitamins and You (1978) by Robert J. Benowicz (Grosset and Dunlap, Inc., 51 Madison Avenue, New York, N.Y. 10010).

The Dieter's Gourmet Cookbook (1979); *Diet for Life* (1980); *New Gourmet Recipes for Dieters* (1981); *The Best of Francine Prince's Diet Gourmet Recipes* (1982)—four books by Francine Prince that represent the best in "new nutrition" cuisine (Cornerstone Library/Simon and Schuster, 1230 Avenue of the Americas, New York, N.Y. 10020).

Eat Right and Stay Healthy (1979) by Dr. Denis Burkitt (Arco Publishing Co., Inc., 219 Park Avenue South, New York, N.Y. 10003).

Permanent Weight Control (1976) by Michael J. Mahoney, Ph.D., and Kathryn Mahoney (W. W. Norton & Co., Inc., 500 Fifth Avenue, New York, N.Y. 10036).

Pure and Simple (1978) by Marilyn Burros (William Morrow & Co., 105 Madison Avenue, New York, N.Y. 10016).

Jane Brody's Nutrition Book (1981) by Jane E. Brody (W. W. Norton & Co., Inc., 500 Fifth Avenue, New York, N.Y. 10036).

Index of Recipes

MEAT-POULTRY-FISH-BEANS GROUP

MILK-CHEESE GROUP

Index

241